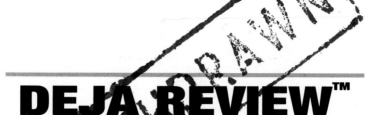

DEJA REVIEW™

Family Medicine

NOTICE

Medicine is an ever-changing science. As new research and clinical experience broaden our knowledge, changes in treatment and drug therapy are required. The authors and the publisher of this work have checked with sources believed to be reliable in their efforts to provide information that is complete and generally in accord with the standards accepted at the time of publication. However, in view of the possibility of human error or changes in medical sciences, neither the authors nor the publisher nor any other party who has been involved in the preparation or publication of this work warrants that the information contained herein is in every respect accurate or complete, and they disclaim all responsibility for any errors or omissions or for the results obtained from use of the information contained in this work. Readers are encouraged to confirm the information contained herein with other sources. For example and in particular, readers are advised to check the product information sheet included in the package of each drug they plan to administer to be certain that the information contained in this work is accurate and that changes have not been made in the recommended dose or in the contraindications for administration. This recommendation is of particular importance in connection with new or infrequently used drugs.

DEJA REVIEW™

Family Medicine

Second Edition

Mayra Perez, MD

Department of Family Medicine
The Methodist Hospital of Houston
Houston, Texas

Winston Liaw, MD, MPH

Assistant Professor
Department of Family Medicine
Virginia Commonwealth University—Fairfax
Fairfax, Virginia

Lindsay K. Botsford, MD

Family Medicine Physician
Kelsey-Seybold Clinic
Houston, Texas

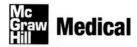

New York   Chicago   San Francisco   Lisbon   London   Madrid   Mexico City
Milan   New Delhi   San Juan   Seoul   Singapore   Sydney   Toronto

Déjà Review™: Family Medicine, Second Edition

Copyright © 2011, 2008 by The McGraw-Hill Companies, Inc. All rights reserved. Printed in the United States of America. Except as permitted under the United States Copyright Act of 1976, no part of this publication may be reproduced or distributed in any form or by any means, or stored in a data base or retrieval system, without the prior written permission of the publisher.

Déjà Review™ is a trademark of The McGraw-Hill Companies, Inc.

1 2 3 4 5 6 7 8 9 0   DOC/DOC   15 14 13 12 11

ISBN 978-0-07-171515-7
MHID 0-07-171515-0

This book was set in Palatino by Glyph International.
The editors were Kirsten Funk and Christine Diedrich.
The production supervisor was Catherine Saggese.
Project management was provided by Tania Andrabi, Glyph International.
RR Donnelley was printer and binder.

This book is printed on acid-free paper.

Library of Congress Cataloging-in-Publication Data

Perez, Mayra.
    Déjà review. Family medicine / Mayra Perez, Winston Liaw, Lindsay K.
Botsford.—2nd ed.
        p. ; cm.—(Deja review)
    Family medicine
    Includes index.
    ISBN-13: 978-0-07-171515-7 (pbk. : alk. paper)
    ISBN-10: 0-07-171515-0 (pbk. : alk. paper)   1. Family medicine—Examinations,
questions, etc.   I. Botsford, Lindsay K.   II. Liaw, Winston. III. Title.   IV. Title:
Family medicine.   V. Series: Deja review.
    [DNLM: 1. Family Practice—Examination Questions.   WB 18.2]
    RC58.P445 2011
    616.0076—dc22
                                                                        2011004682

McGraw-Hill books are available at special quantity discounts to use as premiums and sales promotions, or for use in corporate training programs. To contact a representative please e-mail us at bulksales@mcgraw-hill.com.

To my heroes, my mom and my grandmother;
to John for his patience and unconditional support;
and to my angels, Julia and Marisa
—Mayra Perez

To my parents and grandparents who encouraged me
to never stop learning and supported me along the way;
to my rocks: sis, who never ceases to inspire,
and Eden, my instant happiness
—Winston Liaw

To all my teachers who inspired my curiosity and
passion for learning, to my parents and sisters
for their love and encouragement,
and to John for his patience and support
—Lindsay K. Botsford

Contents

Reviewers

Preface

Family Medicine is challenging and unique because of the broad range of subjects it covers. No book can teach you everything about family medicine, so our intent is to help you identify and learn about the most commonly encountered clinical scenarios in our field, the subjects on which you are most likely to be tested. We recommend browsing the sections at the beginning of the rotation and identifying your strengths and weaknesses. It will give you a good idea of what subject areas to focus on with your preceptor during your rotation. As you become comfortable with certain topics, find the appropriate chapter and test your knowledge. We recommend reading the professional association summaries on hypertension (JNC7), hypercholesterolemia (ATP III), and diabetes (ADA Clinical Practice Recommendations) as early as you can during your rotation. We also recommend using the American Academy of Family Practitioners and United States Preventive Services Task Force websites as key family medicine references.

ORGANIZATION

The *Deja Review* series is a unique resource that has been designed to allow you to review the essential facts and determine your level of knowledge on the subjects tested on your clerkship shelf exams, as well as the United States Medical Licensing Examination (USMLE) Step 2 CK. All concepts are presented in a question and answer format that covers key facts on commonly tested topics during the clerkship.

This question and answer format has several important advantages:

- It provides a rapid, straightforward way for you to assess your strengths and weaknesses.
- Prepares you for "pimping".
- It allows you to efficiently review and commit to memory a large body of information.
- It serves as a quick, last-minute review of high-yield facts.
- Compact, condensed design of the book is conducive to studying on the go.

At the end of the book, you will find clinical vignettes. These vignettes are meant to be representative of the types of questions tested on national licensing exams to help you further evaluate your understanding of the material.

HOW TO USE THIS BOOK

This book is intended to serve as a tool during your family medicine clerkship. Remember, this text is not intended to replace comprehensive textbooks, course packs, or lectures. It is simply intended to serve as a supplement to your studies during your family medicine rotation and throughout your preparation for Step 2 CK. This text was thoroughly reviewed by a number of medical students and interns to represent the core topics tested on shelf examinations. For this reason, we encourage you to begin using this book early in your clinical years to reinforce topics you encounter in the clinic. You may use the book to quiz yourself or classmates on topics covered in recent lectures and clinical case discussions. A bookmark is included so that you can easily cover the answers as you work through each chapter. The compact, condensed design of the book is conducive to studying on the go. Carry it in your white coat pocket so that you can access it during any downtime throughout your busy day.

However you choose to study, we hope you find this resource helpful throughout your preparation for shelf examinations, the USMLE Step 2 CK, and throughout your clinical years.

Mayra Perez
Winston Liaw
Lindsay K. Botsford

SECTION I

Management of Chronic Diseases

CHAPTER 1

Diabetes

What is the mechanism for type I diabetes mellitus (DM)?

Insulin deficiency

What is the mechanism for type II DM?

Insulin resistance

What are the main differences between type I and II DM in terms of age of onset, autoimmunity, body habitus, and risk for ketosis?

Differences between Type I and II Diabetes Mellitus (DM)

	DM I	DM II
Average age of onset	<20 years old	>40 years old[a]
Body habitus	Lean	Obese
Autoimmunity	Yes	No
Risk for ketosis	Yes	Rare

[a]With increasing incidence of childhood obesity, the incidence of DM II is increasing in younger persons.

Which autoantibodies can be positive in type I DM?

Anti-islet cell, antiglutamic acid dehydrogenase antibodies

Does the absence of autoantibodies rule out the diagnosis of type I DM?

No. Some patients with type I DM do not have autoantibodies, and some with type II DM do.

What are some classic presenting symptoms of DM?

Polyuria, polydipsia, unexplained weight loss, blurry vision

How do you diagnose diabetes?   Any one of the following criteria:

Diabetes Diagnostic Criteria

	Fasting blood glucose (FBG), mg/dL[a]	Oral glucose tolerance test (OGTT), mg/dL[b]	Random glucose, mg/dL	Hemoglobin A1 (HbA1c)
Diabetes mellitus	≥126	≥200	≥200 + classic symptoms	≥6.5[c]
Prediabetes	100-125 = Impaired fasting glucose (IFG)	140-199 = Impaired glucose tolerance (IGT)	126-199 → Perform follow-up FBG	
Normal	<100	<140	≤125	<6.5

[a]Fasting = no caloric intake >8 hours
[b]Check glucose 2 hours after a 75-g glucose load.
[c]The test should be performed in a lab using a method that is National Glycohemoglobin Standardization Program certified and standardized to the Diabetes Control and Complications Trial assay.

What do you do after an abnormal test?

Confirm the diagnosis on a subsequent day by using FBG, OGTT, or HbA1c. Patients with glucose ≥200 mg/dL and classic symptoms do not need repeat testing.

What is prediabetes?

Impaired fasting glucose and/or impaired glucose tolerance

What is the clinical implication of prediabetes?

Patients with prediabetes have an increased risk for future development of diabetes mellitus and macrovascular disease. They have a 50% increased risk for myocardial infarction or stroke.

What is the clinical management of a patient with prediabetes?

Address risk factors, measure blood pressure (BP) and serum lipids, and rescreen for diabetes annually.

What behavior changes should you encourage in a patient with prediabetes?

Smoking cessation, weight loss (5%-10%), diet changes, exercise (30 minutes per day, five times per week)

Why is it important to identify patients with prediabetes?

Lifestyle modifications can delay and even prevent progression to diabetes.

What are the three main microvascular complications of diabetes?

1. Retinopathy
2. Nephropathy
3. Neuropathy

What are the three main macrovascular complications of diabetes?

1. Atherosclerosis
2. Cerebrovascular disease
3. Peripheral vascular disease

How frequently should diabetics be seen by an ophthalmologist?

Annually

What is the incidence of retinopathy in patients who have had type II DM for 20 years?

50%-80%

What is usually the first sign of diabetic kidney damage?

Microalbuminuria

What medication can help reduce the risk of diabetic nephropathy?

Angiotensin-converting enzyme inhibitors or angiotension II receptor blockers

What are the different types of diabetic neuropathies?

Peripheral, autonomic, mononeuropathy (eg, cranial nerve palsy)

Describe the manifestations of diabetic peripheral neuropathy?

Symmetric sensory dysfunction, distal sensory loss, paresthesias

How do you test for diabetic peripheral neuropathy?

Place a monofilament at a right angle to the plantar surface of the skin of the foot. Increase the pressure until the monofilament buckles. Ask the patient whether or not he/she felt the pressure from the filament.

How should diabetics care for their feet?

Inspect feet daily for skin cracks and signs of infection between the toes, avoid walking barefoot, ensure shoes fit appropriately.

What should you look for when examining the feet of diabetics?

Skin breaks, early ulcers, decreased pedal pulses, delayed capillary refill, bony deformities

Describe the manifestations of autonomic neuropathy.

Gastroparesis, orthostatic hypotension, impotence, neurogenic bladder

What interventions did the UK Prospective Diabetes Study compare?	Four thousand type II diabetics were assigned to either intensive therapy (sulfonylurea, metformin, and/or insulin) or diet alone.
What did the study show?	• Intensive therapy caused a 1% fall in HbA1c and was associated with a 35% reduction in microvascular endpoints (though most of the benefit was attributable to a decreased need to use photocoagulation for retinopathy) • Metformin (but not sulfonylurea or insulin) decreased mortality independent of blood sugar control • Tight BP control in diabetics reduced mortality
How is HbA1c formed?	Glucose irreversibly attaches to hemoglobin at a rate dependent on blood glucose.
What does HbA1c indirectly measure?	The patient's average glucose level over the preceding 120 days (the life span of RBCs), although it best correlates with average blood glucose over 56-84 days
What will falsely elevate HbA1c?	Any process that decreases RBC turnover (eg, vitamin B_{12}, folate, or iron deficiency)
What will falsely decrease HbA1c?	Any process that increases RBC turnover (eg, hemolysis)
How frequently should HbA1c be checked?	Every 3-4 months until at goal, then every 6 months
What is the goal for HbA1c?	HbA1c <7% (an average blood glucose of 154 mg/dL)
What is the treatment for type I DM?	Insulin replacement
What are the treatments for type II DM?	Weight loss (exercise and American Diabetes Association diet), oral hypoglycemic medications (see table on next page), exogenous insulin

Oral Hypoglycemic Medications

	Mechanism of Action	Side Effects/Disadvantages	Comments
Biguanides (metformin)	Decrease hepatic glucose production	Lactic acidosis especially in patients with renal insufficiency (stop medication if the creatinine is >1.5 mg/dL in men or 1.4 mg/dL in women), diarrhea, and nausea	Can cause weight stabilization/reduction, low risk of hypoglycemia, generic version is inexpensive
Sulfonylureas (eg, glimepiride, glyburide, glipizide)	Increase insulin secretion by pancreatic beta cells	High risk of hypoglycemia, weight gain	Rapid reduction of fasting plasma glucose, generics are inexpensive
Thiazolidinediones (eg, rosiglitazone, pioglitazone)	Increase insulin sensitivity in muscle and fat cells	Liver toxicity and fluid retention (caution in patients with congestive heart failure), rosiglitazone has a black box warning for its increased risk of myocardial infarctions	Low risk of hypoglycemia

(Continued)

Oral Hypoglycemic Medications (Continued)

	Mechanism of Action	Side Effects/Disadvantages	Comments
GLP-1 analogs (exenatide) and DPP-IV inhibitors[a] **(sitagliptin)**	GLP-1 enhances insulin secretion, slows gastric emptying, and suppresses postprandial glucagon. DPP-IV *inactivates* GLP-1.	Nausea which is associated with weight loss (for GLP-1 analogs only)	Low risk of hypoglycemia
Alpha-glucosidase inhibitors (eg, acarbose and miglitol)	Inhibit intestinal conversion of carbohydrates to monosaccharides	Diarrhea and flatulence	Low risk of hypoglycemia
Meglitinides (repaglinide and nateglinide)	Taken just prior to a meal, stimulate insulin secretion by pancreatic beta cells	Expensive and requires frequent dosing	Helpful for patients with high postprandial glucose, meal-adjusted dosing, low risk of hypoglycemia

[a]GLP-1: glucagon-like peptide, DPP-IV: dipeptidyl peptidase IV

Sulfonylureas and metformin can each decrease fasting glucose by what percentage?

20%

Sulfonylureas and metformin can each decrease HbA1c by what percentage?

1%-2%

After 3 years of monotherapy, what percentage of patients will require the addition of a second medication for glycemic control?

50%

What is the BP goal for diabetics?

SBP <130 mm Hg and DBP <80 mm Hg

Why is BP control important in diabetics?

A 10-mm Hg reduction in systolic BP is associated with a 12% risk reduction in any diabetes-related complication.

What is the LDL goal for diabetics?

LDL <100 mg/dL

In addition to cholesterol and BP control, what other interventions are recommended for diabetics to reduce macrovascular complications?

Smoking cessation, daily aspirin if the risk of developing coronary artery disease over the next 10 years is >10%

Which vaccines should be given to diabetics?

Yearly influenza vaccine, pneumonia vaccine (repeat dose after age 65 if the first dose was given prior to age 65 and was given 5 years previously)

Name the different types of insulin and their approximate duration of action.

The Onset, Peak, and Duration of Insulin Preparations

	Onset (hours)	Peak (hours)	Duration (hours)
Fast-acting			
Lispro	0.25-0.5	0.5-2.5	<5
Regular insulin	0.5	2-4	5-7
Intermediate-acting			
NPH (neutral protamine hagedorn)	1-2	6-10	14-24
Long-acting			
Ultralente	3-4	No peak	~24
Glargine (lantus)	3-4	No peak	~24

What is the definition of the metabolic syndrome according to the National Cholesterol Education Program/Adult Treatment Panel III?

Any three of the following:
1. Abdominal obesity (waist circumference in men >40 in, women >35 in)
2. Serum triglycerides ≥150 mg/dL or drug treatment for elevated triglycerides
3. Serum high-density lipoprotein (HDL) cholesterol <40 mg/dL in men and <50 mg/dL in women or drug treatment for low HDL
4. BP ≥130/85 mm Hg or drug treatment for elevated BP
5. Fasting plasma glucose (FPG) ≥100 mg/dL or drug treatment for elevated blood glucose

What are the clinical implications of having the metabolic syndrome?

Increased risk of developing diabetes and cardiovascular disease

What is the body mass index (BMI) measurement?

An indirect approximation of body fat

How is BMI calculated?

([Weight in lbs.]/[height in in.]^2) × 703

or

(Weight in kgs.)/(height in m.)^2

Which BMI level represents being overweight?

Between 25 and 29.9

Which BMI level represents being obese?

≥30

In what situation does BMI overestimate body fat?

A person with a higher than average percentage of muscle mass

Which diseases of the exocrine pancreas can cause diabetes?

Cystic fibrosis, hemochromatosis, chronic pancreatitis

Which endocrinopathies can cause diabetes?

Any increase in hormones that inhibit insulin: Cushing (cortisol), glucagonoma (glucagon), pheochromocytoma (epinephrine), acromegaly (growth hormone)

What is diabetic ketoacidosis (DKA)?

A medical emergency where insulin deficiency leads to hyperglycemia, electrolyte disturbances, ketonemia, and metabolic acidosis

How does the insulin deficiency precipitate DKA?

In insulin deficiency, the liver breaks down lipids into ketone bodies resulting in a decrease in blood pH (serum ketones + acidosis).

What can precipitate DKA?

I's: Infection, Infarction (cardiac, cerebral, mesenteric), Insulin (prescription dose is too low, patient is noncompliant), Intraabdominal process (pancreatitis), Intoxication (alcohol), Idiopathic. Also consider physical stress and drugs (eg, glucocorticoids, second-generation antipsychotics).

How do you categorize the acid-base abnormality in DKA?

Anion gap metabolic acidosis with compensatory respiratory alkalosis

What is Kussmaul breathing?

Rapid, deep breathing to help increase CO_2 excretion and correct the underlying acidosis in DKA

A patient with DKA can have what odor to their breath?

Fruity, acetone odor

What is the treatment of DKA?

Aggressive IV fluids, IV insulin, acid-base and electrolyte management (potassium, phosphorus)

When can you transition the patient from IV insulin to subcutaneous insulin?

When the anion gap has resolved and the bicarbonate level approaches normal

What are the diagnostic criteria for hyperosmolar hyperglycemia state (HHS)?

Plasma glucose >600 mg/dL, arterial pH >7.3, serum bicarbonate >18 mEq/L, effective serum osmolality >320 mOsm/kg, minimal ketones in serum and urine

How do you manage HHS?

Aggressive IV fluids, IV insulin, correction of electrolyte abnormalities (such as potassium depletion), monitoring of urine output and mental status

What percentage of patients with HHS also present with neurologic abnormalities such as coma?

25%-50%. Neurologic changes occur in patients with effective plasma osmolalities above 320 mOsm/kg.

CHAPTER 2

Cardiovascular Disease

HYPERTENSION

What is normal blood pressure (BP) in adults (units = mm Hg)?

Systolic blood pressure (SBP) <120 mm Hg *and* diastolic blood pressure (DBP) <80 mm Hg

What is prehypertension?

Stage 1 hypertension (HTN)?

SBP of 120-139 mm Hg *or* DBP of 80-89 mm Hg

Stage 2 HTN?

SBP of 140-159 mm Hg *or* DBP of 90-99 mm Hg

SBP ≥160 mm Hg *or* DBP ≥100 mm Hg

List the five important environmental causal factors for primary HTN.

1. Excessive weight
2. Sedentary lifestyle
3. Excessive sodium intake
4. Inadequate intake of fruits, vegetables, and potassium
5. Excessive alcohol intake

How do you diagnose HTN?

Two or more properly measured elevated BPs on each of two or more office visits

A patient with HTN typically has NO symptoms. True or false?

True. However, evidence of end-organ damage may appear as the disease progresses. Assess symptoms at each visit: chest pain, shortness of breath, abdominal pain, oliguria, headache, dizziness/syncope, vision changes.

What are the goals of the history and physical examination for a patient with HTN?

Assess adequacy of disease management and factors that affect prognosis (medications, lifestyle, etc), identify co-morbidities, assess overall cardiovascular disease (CVD) risk, assess the extent of end-organ damage, rule out secondary causes of HTN

What physical examination components are especially important to document in an initial assessment of patients with HTN?

Vital signs (including BP in all extremities and body mass index), cardiopulmonary exam, neck exam (thyroid, carotids), optic fundi, abdominal exam (check for aneurysm, renal/femoral bruits, organomegaly), extremities (pulses, check for edema), neurologic exam

Effectively controlling BP reduces patient morbidity and mortality by decreasing the incidence of what medical conditions?

CVD, transient ischemic attack/stroke, aneurysms, dementia, retinopathy, chronic kidney disease (CKD)

BP control decreases the incidence of what specific cardiovascular diseases?

Heart failure, left ventricular hypertrophy, cardiomyopathy, myocardial infarction, peripheral vascular disease

The relationship between elevated BP and CVD is independent of other risk factors for CVD. True or false?

True

Beginning at a BP of 115/75 mm Hg, each incremental increase in BP of 20/10 mm Hg doubles the risk of CVD. True or false?

True

What tests should be performed in patients with HTN before initiating therapy?

EKG, blood glucose and hematocrit, serum potassium and calcium, creatinine (or calculated GFR), fasting lipid profile, urinalysis, urine albumin excretion, or albumin to creatinine ratio (optional)

How often should potassium and creatinine be checked thereafter?

Twice a year (additional periodic labs are based on co-morbidities)

How do you measure albumin in the urine?

Spot urine albumin to urine creatinine ratio (24-hour urine collection is not necessary)

What conditions warrant screening for albuminuria annually in patients with HTN?

Patients with HTN who also have diabetes or kidney disease

Uncontrolled SBP can accelerate the decline of GFR by as much as 4-8 mL/min per year. True or false?

True

Define the goal of BP management in patients without complicated HTN.	BP <140/90 mm Hg
Define the goal for BP management in patients with a treatment-altering comorbidity.	BP <130/80 mm Hg
Name these treatment-altering co-morbidities.	CKD, diabetes, CVD
Most people will reach their DBP goal when the SBP goal is achieved, so therapy should focus on lowering the SBP. True or false?	True
Why is it important to identify patients with prehypertension?	Patients in this category are at twice the risk of developing overt HTN than those with normal BPs.
In the absence of co-morbidities, are prehypertensive patients candidates for drug therapy?	No, but it is important to intervene early and educate the patient on healthy lifestyle modifications.
Name lifestyle modifications for prehypertension and HTN.	1. Weight loss 2. DASH diet 3. Regular aerobic exercise 4. Reduced alcohol intake 5. Smoking cessation
What does DASH stand for?	Dietary Approaches to Stop Hypertension
Describe the DASH diet.	1. Rich in fruits, vegetables, and dairy products 2. Low in cholesterol and saturated and total fat 3. Rich in potassium and calcium 4. Less than 2.4 g (preferably 1.6 g) of sodium per day
Following the 1.6 g sodium DASH diet has similar effects to single-drug therapy. True or false?	True
Unless there is a compelling indication to start another medication, what drug should be initiated in cases of uncomplicated stage 1 HTN?	Low-dose thiazide diuretic

Thiazide diuretics are usually first line treatment, but for the following compelling indications, what anti-hypertensives are acceptable alternatives to thiazides or should be used in conjunction with a thiazide?

Heart failure

Beta-blocker (BB), angiotensin-converting enzyme inhibitor (ACEI), angiotensin receptor blocker (ARB), aldosterone antagonist

Post-myocardial infarction

BB, ACEI, aldosterone antagonist

High risk of coronary artery disease

BB, ACEI, calcium-channel blocker (CCB)

Diabetes mellitus

BB, ACEI, ARB, CCB

Chronic kidney disease

ACEI or ARB

Recurrent stroke

ACEI

What are the contraindications to beta-blocker use?

Severe reactive airway disease, uncompensated heart failure, severe peripheral arterial disease, bradycardia or hypotension, high-grade AV block, or sick sinus syndrome

When should you initiate treatment with *two* anti-hypertensive agents?

Patient's BP is >20/10 mm Hg than the target BP, even if current drug dosage is not maxed out.

About what percentage of HTN patients can have controlled BP on only one medication?

30%

After initiation of antihypertensive drug therapy, how often should patients follow up for medication adjustments?

Monthly, until BP goal is reached (more often if patient has stage 2 HTN or co-morbidities)

Once desired BP is achieved, approximately how often should patients follow up?

Every 3-6 months

When should ambulatory BP monitoring be considered?

Wide variation in self-reported BP readings; evaluation of White Coat HTN; assessment of drug effectiveness, side effects, or resistance

What percent of patients have no direct identifiable cause of their HTN?	90%-95%
What term is used to describe this type of HTN?	Primary (essential) hypertension
What percent of patients have secondary HTN (*do* have an identifiable cause)?	5%-10%
What is the most common cause of secondary HTN?	Renovascular hypertension
What processes cause renovascular HTN?	Atherosclerotic renal artery stenosis, fibromuscular dysplasia, vasculitis
In general, which is most common in older men?	Atherosclerotic renal artery stenosis
Younger women?	Fibromuscular dysplasia

For the following case scenarios, list the most likely cause of secondary HTN.

Abdominal bruit on physical examination	Renovascular hypertension
Headache, sweating, and palpitations with periods of acute BP elevations	Pheochromocytoma
Diminished or delayed peripheral pulses, a bruit heard over the back, higher SBP in the upper extremities than in the lower extremities	Aortic coarctation
Truncal obesity, glucose intolerance, and abdominal striae	Cushing syndrome
Therapy with ACEI or ARB precipitates acute renal failure	Bilateral renal artery stenosis

How do you evaluate the following causes of secondary HTN?

Obstructive sleep apnea (OSA)

Sleep study with O_2 saturation

Drug-induced or drug-related HTN

Review patient's medications and identify potential BP elevators (eg, non-steroidal anti-inflammatory drugs, steroids, estrogens), ask patient about current or recent use of herbal remedies, alcohol, illicit drugs, nicotine.

Primary aldosteronism or other mineralocorticoid excess state

24-hour urine aldosterone level or specific measurements of other mineralocorticoids

Renovascular disease

Doppler flow study or magnetic resonance angiography

Cushing syndrome or other steroid excess

Dexamethasone suppression test

Pheochromocytoma

24-hour urinary catecholamines

Coarctation of the aorta

Computed tomography angiography

Thyroid or parathyroid disease

Thyroid stimulating hormone (TSH) and serum parathyroid hormone

How common is hypertension among patients with OSA?

50% of patients with OSA have HTN.

LIPID LOWERING

When hypercholesterolemia is identified, what further laboratory workup is indicated?

Fasting blood glucose, TSH, liver function tests (LFTs), creatinine

The primary target of cholesterol lowering therapy is low-density lipoprotein (LDL). How is the LDL goal established?

By determining the patient's risk of having a coronary heart disease (CHD) event sometime in the next 10 years

List CHD risk factors.

HTN, high-density lipoprotein (HDL) <40 mg/dL, smoking, male >45 years old, female >55 years old, family history of early CHD (first-degree male with CHD <55 years old, first-degree female with CHD <65 years old)

What HDL level is considered a negative risk factor and may be counted as a "minus one" toward the overall number of CHD risk factors?

HDL >60 mg/dL

What lifestyle modifications can increase HDL?

Increased aerobic activity and moderate alcohol consumption (1-2 drinks per day)

List CHD equivalents.

1. Diabetes mellitus
2. Peripheral artery disease
3. Any combination of risk factors leading to a cumulative 10-year CHD risk of over 20% (as determined by a risk calculator—widely available, including at http://hp2010.nhlbihin.net/atpiii/calculator.asp)
4. Symptomatic carotid artery disease
5. Abdominal aortic aneurysm

Fill in the blank: someone with known CHD or a CHD equivalent has a ___% risk of having another CHD event sometime in the next 10 years.

>20

What lifestyle modifications can lower LDL?

1. Dietary modifications
2. Increased physical activity
3. Smoking cessation
4. Weight loss

Lifestyle changes and medical therapy should be implemented when LDL reaches what level (>100 mg/dL, >130 mg/dL, >160 mg/dL)?

Refer to the table below:

LDL Treatment Guidelines

Category	LDL to Start Lifestyle Change, Mg/Dl	LDL to Consider Drug Therapy, mg/dL
CHD, risk equivalent, or 10-year risk >20%	≥100	≥130 (100-129 drug therapy optional)
2 risk factors, with 10-year risk 10%-20%	≥130	≥130
2 risk factors, with 10-year risk <10%	≥130	≥160
0-1 risk factors	≥160	≥190 (160-189 drug therapy optional)

To lower cholesterol levels, what dietary modifications should be made in regards to fat intake?

1. Total dietary fat should be less than 35% of total caloric intake (<10% polyunsaturated fat, <7% saturated fat).
2. Cholesterol intake less than 200 mg/day.

What is the LDL goal for patients with CHD or a CHD equivalent?

LDL <100 mg/dL

What is the LDL goal for patients with 0-1 risk factor(s) and no CHD or a CHD equivalent?

LDL <160 mg/dL

LDL <70 is an optional goal for which subset of patients?

Very high-risk patients (recent myocardial infarction, metabolic syndrome, CVD with diabetes or severe or poorly controlled risk factors such as smoking)

How long after initial lifestyle modifications and/or medical therapy is started should lipids be rechecked?

6 weeks

What class of drugs represents the current first line pharmacotherapy in the lowering of LDL?

Statins

What is the mechanism of action of statins?

Inhibit HMG-CoA reductase (enzyme in the pathway that produces cholesterol)

Statins lower LDL levels by what percentage?

20%-40%

Statins increase HDL by what percentage?

5%-15%

What are the major contraindications to statin use?

Acute or chronic liver disease, concomitant use of certain drugs (eg, macrolides, alcohol), history of serious adverse effects with statins (eg, rhabdomyolysis)

What percentage of patients on a statin will experience myalgias as a side effect?

5%

What fat-soluble substance found in some foods (highest in meat and fish) that is also available as a vitamin supplement may be used to reduce myalgia symptoms in many patients?

Coenzyme Q10 (ubiquinone): 100 mg PO daily as a supplement dose

What percentage of patients on a statin will develop rhabdomyolysis?

0.1%

What are the symptoms of rhabdomyolysis (should prompt patient to stop statin immediately)?

Severe myalgias, muscle weakness, dark urine

What are the risk factors for statin-induced myopathy?

Concurrent use of a fibric acid derivative (especially gemfibrozil), older age, female gender, low weight, acute physical stress

If a patient is on a statin, how often should you monitor liver transaminases (assuming the patient has no history of chronic liver disease)?

Check at baseline (after statin initiation or dose change) and assuming transaminases remain normal, recheck them in 6-12 weeks, 3 months, and thereafter every 6-12 months. If transaminases are elevated, increase testing frequency to as often as clinically necessary.

If a patient has no prior history of liver disease and the patient's liver transaminases increase with statin treatment, the statin should be discontinued when the transaminases reach what level?

Three times greater than the baseline levels

If a patient has a history of chronic liver disease and the patient's liver transaminases increase with statin treatment, the statin should be discontinued when the transaminases reach what level?

Two times greater than the baseline levels

Rank the following statins in order from least to most potent: atorvastatin, fluvastatin, lovastatin, pravastatin, rosuvastatin, simvastatin.

Fluvastatin, pravastatin, lovastatin, simvastatin, atorvastatin, rosuvastatin

Of these statins, which one is NOT metabolized by the CYP 450 system and thus is less likely to cause drug interactions?

Pravastatin (greater renal metabolism)

Of these statins, which ones are more favorable for usage in patients with renal impairment?

Atorvastatin and fluvastatin

What drugs should be considered for the treatment of hypertriglyceridemia?	Fibric acid derivatives (fibrates), niacin, fish oil supplements (>3 g per day)
What are the absolute contraindications to use of fibrates?	Pre-existing gallstones, hepatic or renal disease

CARDIOMYOPATHY

List the three types of cardiomyopathy.	1. Dilated cardiomyopathy (DCM) 2. Restrictive cardiomyopathy (RCM) 3. Hypertrophic cardiomyopathy (HCM)
Describe DCM.	Typically involves LV dilation and systolic dysfunction (but may involve four-chamber dilation). Therapy is directed at treating systolic dysfunction.
List some conditions that can lead to DCM.	Alcohol, atrial flutter, atrial fibrillation, thyroid dysfunction, pregnancy, adenovirus, HIV, SLE, cocaine, Beriberi (vitamin B1 deficiency)
DCM is diagnosed with what imaging modality?	Echocardiography
Describe RCM.	Diastolic dysfunction without evidence of dilation or hypertrophy of the left ventricle. Therapy is directed at treating diastolic dysfunction.
List some conditions that can lead to RCM.	Amyloidosis, sarcoidosis, glycogen storage diseases, hemochromatosis, idiopathic RCM
How is RCM evaluated?	Echocardiography (to reveal small ventricles and systolic abnormality in the presence of diastolic dysfunction)
What is the most common cause of sudden cardiac death in young athletes?	Hypertrophic cardiomyopathy
Describe HCM.	A genetic disease characterized by hypertrophy of the ventricles (caused by a cardiac sarcomere defect)

What disease states fall under this general category?	Hypertrophic obstructive cardiomyopathy (HOCM), asymmetric septal hypertrophy (ASH), idiopathic hypertrophic subaortic stenosis (IHSS)
How is HCM diagnosed?	EKG to demonstrate left axis deviation and left ventricular hypertrophy, echocardiography to show ventricular thickening
What classes of drugs are typically used to treat HCM?	Calcium-channel blockers and beta-blockers
When should surgical treatment for HCM be considered?	LV outflow tract obstruction is inadequately controlled by medical management

VALVULAR DISEASE

What is a normal aortic valve area?	Between 3 and 4 cm^2 in adults
What is the aortic valve area in critical aortic stenosis (AS)?	<0.8 cm^2
List the three most common causes of AS.	1. Bicuspid aortic valve 2. Degenerative changes associated with the aging process (primarily sclerosis) 3. Rheumatic fever
What are the symptoms of AS?	Angina, congestive heart failure symptoms, syncope
Describe the typical signs of AS.	Normal to low BP, "parvus et tardus" (a weak and slow carotid pulse that often rises slowly and with a shudder), crescendo-decrescendo murmur at the right second intercostal space that radiates to the neck
How should AS be treated if it is asymptomatic?	No intervention is indicated.
How should the disease be managed once symptoms begin?	Surgery

HEART FAILURE

What is heart failure (HF)?

The heart's ability to pump is inadequate and unable to maintain the body's circulatory needs.

What are the two types of HF?

Systolic dysfunction and diastolic dysfunction

Describe systolic dysfunction.

Dilated left ventricle with impaired ability to contract

Describe diastolic dysfunction.

Left ventricle appears normal but has impaired ability to relax and fill.

What is a normal ejection fraction (EF)?

>55%

Which has a normal EF, systolic or diastolic HF?

Diastolic

Describe the role of anti-hypertensives in the treatment of HF.

Decrease afterload so the heart pumps against less resistance

How does chronic atrial fibrillation (AF) affect a patient with HF?

Tachycardia and decreased atrial contraction worsens left ventricle filling, so AF rate control is important.

What agents should be used to achieve AF rate control?

BB, CCB

What is BNP?

Brain natriuretic peptide—released from heart ventricle myocytes when they are stretched

What is a normal BNP level?

<100 pg/mL

What is the BNP level seen in HF?

>500 pg/mL (between 100 and 500 pg/mL is inconclusive)

What are some common symptoms of left-sided HF?

Weakness and dyspnea with exertion (sometimes even at rest); paroxysmal nocturnal dyspnea; orthopnea; cough; wheezing; pink, frothy sputum

What are some physical findings of left-sided HF?

Bilateral pulmonary crackles (rales), S3 gallop, displaced PMI

What are some common symptoms of right-sided HF?	Abdominal pain and bloating, nausea and vomiting, anorexia, constipation
What are some physical findings of right-sided HF?	Peripheral edema, jugular venous distention, hepatosplenomegaly, hepatojugular reflux, ascites
What are some common chest x-ray findings found in HF patients?	Pleural effusions, pulmonary edema, cephalization of pulmonary vessels, cardiomegaly (cardiothoracic ratio >50%)
List cardiovascular diseases that lead to HF.	Ischemic heart disease, HTN, valvular disease, cardiac rhythm disorders, cardiomyopathies
Describe the mechanisms by which ischemic heart disease may cause HF.	1. Chronic ischemia causes sub-optimal myocardial function. 2. Previous MI leading to left ventricular dysfunction and subsequent remodeling.
What therapeutic strategies should be applied to HF patients with ischemic heart disease?	Medical treatment for angina, direct efforts to modify cardiac risk factors, consideration of surgery (stenting, angioplasty, coronary artery bypass grafting)
List the recommended lifestyle modifications for HF patients.	Dietary salt limitation, exercise, weight loss, alcohol/smoking cessation
What class of medication is used to treat fluid overload in both the acute and chronic settings?	Diuretics (usually loop diuretic such as furosemide)
In the setting of HF, which antihypertensives have been shown to increase patient survival?	BB (eg, carvedilol, metoprolol suceinate), ACEI, ARB, spironolactone
How have BBs and ACEIs specifically been shown to improve survival?	By reducing heart remodeling and decreasing sympathetic tone (less stress on the heart)
What medications should be initiated for secondary prevention of further cardiovascular events?	Statin and aspirin

What additional medication combination may be of benefit to African American patients with HF?	Hydralazine combined with nitrates
What general medical conditions may lead to HF?	Systemic lupus erythematous (SLE), hemochromatosis, sarcoidosis, cocaine abuse, alcohol abuse
What inflammatory disease is a significant cause of HF?	Myocarditis
List some causes of myocarditis.	Coxsackie B, influenza, adenovirus, rheumatic fever, HIV, Chagas disease, Lyme disease
What lab findings may be abnormal in these patients?	Erythrocyte sedimentation rate elevation, creatinine kinase/troponin elevation during the acute phase, T-wave inversion or ST elevation on EKG
What are some common causes of acute exacerbations of HF?	Infection, anemia, acute myocardial infarction, dietary indiscretions (high salt or water intake)
How do you manage new onset or acute exacerbation of HF requiring hospitalization?	Place patient on telemetry, give IV diuretics, monitor fluid balance and electrolytes closely, administer oxygen, control co-morbidities (especially HTN), evaluate precipitating causes of HF.
How do you evaluate precipitating causes?	Echocardiogram, EKG, chest x-ray (CXR), blood tests
What blood tests should you order in the setting of acute onset of HF?	Complete blood count, basic metabolic panel, liver function tests, cardiac enzymes

STROKE

What is the most common cause of neurologic disability and the third leading cause of death in the United States?	Stroke

What is a transient ischemic attack (TIA)?

It is an ischemia-induced focal neurologic deficit lasting less than 24 hours (usually <1 hour).

What are common signs and symptoms of a TIA?

Ipsilateral blindness (amaurosis fugax), unilateral hemiplegia, hemiparesis, weakness

Why is a TIA important to diagnose?

May be a precursor to stroke

What are the two kinds of strokes?

Ischemic and hemorrhagic

Which type is more common?

Ischemic (about 80%)

What causes an ischemic stroke?

A thrombus or an embolus

What causes a hemorrhagic stroke?

Intracerebral hemorrhage

What is the most common cause of hemorrhagic stroke?

Hypertension

What are other causes of strokes?

Coagulopathy, septic embolus from endocarditis, sickle cell disease, ruptured aneurysm, arteriovenous malformation, malignancy

What are the signs and symptoms of stroke?

Severe headache, vomiting, mental status changes, nuchal rigidity, hemisensory loss, hemiparesis, amaurosis fugax, aphasia, ataxia

What is the initial imaging study you should order if you suspect a stroke?

CT scan of the head without contrast

According to the American Heart Association (AHA)/American Stroke Association (ASA) guidelines, what other diagnostic tests should be performed to evaluate a suspected stroke or TIA?

Magnetic resonance imaging, echocardiogram, EKG, noninvasive imaging of the cervicocephalic vessels

What are the noninvasive options for imaging the cervicocephalic vessels?

Carotid dopplers, magnetic resonance angiography, CT angiography

When can thrombolysis with tissue-plasminogen activator (tPA) be used in a patient with a confirmed ischemic stroke?

The patient presents within the first three hours of onset of symptoms and meets strict criteria for its use.

What are the contraindications of tPA?	Uncontrolled HTN, intracranial pathology (eg, bleeding, neoplasm, arteriovenous malformation), recent major surgery, recent serious head trauma, recent stroke, seizure at the onset of the stroke, high risk of bleeding (eg, heparin within last 48 hours, abnormal partial thromboplastin time, platelets <100,000)
According to the AHA/ASA and the American College of Chest Physicians guidelines, which antiplatelet agents can be used for secondary ischemic stroke prevention?	Aspirin 50-325 mg PO once daily, clopidogrel 75 mg PO once daily, or extended-release dipyridamole 200 mg/ 25 mg aspirin PO two times daily.
Does aspirin plus clopidogrel offer greater benefit than either medication alone?	No

PEDIATRIC CARDIOLOGY

What is the main concern if an infant tires easily (sweating, heavy breathing) while eating?	Possible presence of a congenital heart defect
What causes the sound of a murmur?	Turbulent blood flow
Name five innocent murmurs of childhood.	1. Still 2. Peripheral pulmonic stenosis (PPS) 3. Carotid innominate bruit 4. Venous hum 5. Pulmonary outflow murmur
What does Still murmur sound like?	Musical, twangy, like a rubber band loudest at the apex
Where does the PPS radiate?	It is an ejection murmur that radiates to the axilla and backs.
When does PPS disappear?	Between 6 and 12 months

What is a PDA?

Patent ductus arteriosus (connection remains between the aorta and pulmonary artery)

What does the murmur sound like?

A continuous machine-like murmur

When does the ductus usually close?

Early in the neonatal period

In order, what are the most common congenital cardiac defects?

Ventral septal defect (VSD), pulmonary stenosis, atrial septal defect (ASD), coarctation of the aorta

Why might the murmur of VSD not be appreciable on the first day of life?

High PA pressures on day one may diminish left to right shunting

What physical examination findings help rule out a diagnosis of coarctation of the aorta?

Strong equal palpable femoral pulses, equal upper and lower extremity BP, well-perfused lower extremities

What are the congenitally acquired *cyanotic* heart abnormalities?

Tetralogy of Fallot, transposition of the great vessels, truncus arteriosus, total anomalous pulmonary venous return, tricuspid atresia

Acyanotic?

VSD, ASD, patent ductus arteriosus (PDA)

What are the four anomalies of Tetralogy of Fallot?

Overriding aorta, right ventricular hypertrophy, ventricular septal defect, right ventricular outflow tract obstruction

Describe transposition of the great vessels.

The aorta arises from the right ventricle carrying non-oxigenized blood to the systemic circulation. The pulmonary artery arises from the left ventricle carrying oxygenated blood to the lungs.

What is truncus arteriosus?

A single large vessel (instead of a pulmonary artery and aorta) emerges from the ventricles, usually overriding a VSD.

Besides congential heart disease, what are the other causes of cyanosis in the newborn?

Intrinsic pulmonary disease and central nervous system depression

CHAPTER 3

Chronic Kidney Disease

The kidneys are responsible for what physiologic and chemical functions?

- Rid body of waste products and excess water in the form of urine
- Regulate acid-base and electrolyte balance
- Produce erythropoietin
- Help control blood pressure (BP) through the renin-angiotensin system
- Remove excess phosphorus from the blood
- Convert D3 into calcitriol (active vitamin D)

Renal function, as measured by the glomerular filtration rate (GFR), normally begins to deteriorate in the third or fourth decade of life. True or false?

True (and by the sixth decade, GFR declines by 1-2 mL/min per year)

What is chronic kidney disease (CKD)?

Decreased kidney function as evidenced by decreased GFR and/or persistent albuminuria

The continuum of CKD is divided into five stages based on the rate of what process?

Glomerular filtration

What is normal GFR and what is GFR at the five stages of CKD?

Stage	GFR (mL/min/1.73 m^2)
Normal	>90
1	>90
2	60-89
3	30-59
4	15-29
5	<15 (or the patient is on dialysis)

A patient will usually require dialysis when his/her GFR decreases to what level?

$<15 \text{ mL/min/1.73 m}^2$

Several patients all with the same creatinine level can have different GFRs based on what personal characteristics?

Age, gender, race, body weight

What two equations can be used to calculate GFR?

MDRD (Modification of Diet in Renal Disease) or Cockcroft-Gault (readily available on the Internet, including at http://www.nephron.com)

It is necessary to obtain a 24-hour urine collection in order to calculate urine albumin excretion. True or false?

False. A spot urine albumin to creatinine ratio is adequate and the patient is much more likely to comply with obtaining the test.

What is the equation by which a spot urine albumin to creatinine ratio estimates 24-hour urine albumin excretion?

Urine albumin (mg/dL)/Urine creatinine (g/dL) = Urine albumin to creatinine ratio (UACR). The UACR is approximately equal to the albumin excretion in mg/day.

What is albuminuria?

Abnormally high urinary albumin excretion (UACR is >30 mg/g)

What is range of UACR for microalbuminuria?

Between 30 and 300 mg/g

What are the two most common causes of CKD in American adults?

Diabetes mellitus (DM) and hypertension (HTN)

Under what conditions should patients with these diseases have their urine albumin excretion assessed annually in order to diagnose and monitor CKD?

Patients who have had type I DM for more than 5 years, all patients with type II DM starting at the time of diagnosis, or patients with HTN who also have DM or kidney disease

Before diagnosing CKD, acute renal insufficiency/failure should be ruled out. What are some reversible causes of acute kidney disease?

Volume depletion, urinary outlet obstruction, drug side effects or toxicity

What is the leading cause of death in patients with CKD?

Cardiovascular disease (especially stroke)

What is the target BP for patients with CKD?

$<130/80$ mm Hg (preferably $<125/75$ mm Hg)

What classes of antihypertensives are first-line agents for treatment of high BP in patients with CKD?

Renin-angiotension system antagonists (angiotensin-converting enzyme inhibitors or angiotensin receptor blocker) and thiazide diuretics

Reduced sodium intake is especially important in hypertensive patients with CKD because sodium control is altered. What is the recommended daily intake of sodium in CKD patients?

2300 mg or less

CKD patients should limit their protein intake to what amount per day?

Nondiabetic: 0.8 g/kg

Diabetic: 0.8-1.0 g/kg

In patients with DM and CKD who are on insulin, why is it sometimes necessary to decrease their insulin dose even when their DM is not necessarily improving?

Worsening kidney function may decrease the breakdown of insulin (partially metabolized in the kidney) and lead to hypoglycemia.

What is the main lab value by which nutritional status is monitored in patients with CKD?

Albumin

What is the main mechanism by which CKD causes anemia of chronic disease?

Kidneys produce less erythropoietin → decreased production of red blood cells

What is the general pathophysiology behind renal osteodystrophy?

In CKD, the normal regulation of calcium and phosphorus mediated by vitamin D and parathyroid hormone goes awry and causes bone fragility, pain, and deformation.

When a patient has mineral and hormone disorders resulting from CKD what interventions may help to prevent the development/worsening of renal osteodystrophy?

Diet (decreased oral intake of phosphorus, increased calcium and vitamin D), dialysis, medication (phosphate binders), surgery (parathyroidectomy)

CHAPTER 4

Thyroid Disease

HYPOTHYROIDISM

For the following systems, describe the clinical manifestations of hypothyroidism.

Dermatologic

Decreased blood flow leads to cool skin, coarse hair, and brittle nails. Accumulation of glycosaminoglycans in interstitial spaces causes nonpitting edema (myxedema).

Cardiovascular

Decreased heart rate and contractility → decreased cardiac output → dyspnea on exertion.

Gastrointestinal

Decreased motility leads to constipation

Hematologic

Normocytic anemia

Reproductive

Amenorrhea, menorrhagia, decreased fertility

Neurologic

Carpal tunnel syndrome and delayed deep tendon reflexes

Metabolic

Increased cholesterol and triglycerides, decreased free water clearance leads to hyponatremia, decreased basal metabolic rate → weight gain

What is cretinism?

Congenital hypothyroidism causing mental retardation and impaired growth

Interpret these lab findings.

Low free T4 and high TSH

Overt hypothyroidism

Normal free T4 and high TSH

Subclinical hypothyroidism

Low free T4 and low TSH

Secondary hypothyroidism (rare)

What are some of the conditions that can cause secondary hypothyroidism?

Pituitary macroadenoma, Sheehan syndrome (pituitary infarct secondary to postpartum hemorrhage)

What is the most common cause of hypothyroidism?

Hashimoto thyroiditis (chronic autoimmune thyroiditis)

Which autoantibodies mediate destruction of thyroid tissue in Hashimoto thyroiditis?

Antithyroglobulin and antithyroid peroxidase antibodies

What are risk factors for developing Hashimoto thyroiditis?

Female gender, family history of autoimmune disorders

What are the iatrogenic causes of hypothyroidism?

Thyroidectomy, external radiation therapy, radioiodine therapy

What medications can cause hypothyroidism?

Lithium, amiodarone, interferon alpha, interleukin 2

Iodine deficiency can cause hypothyroidism. True or false?

True. Less than 100 mcg of iodine per day increases the risk of hypothyroidism.

Iodine excess can cause hypothyroidism. True or false?

True. Excess iodine can inhibit the organification of T4 and T3 (Wolff-Chaikoff effect).

What percentage of patients with subclinical hypothyroidism progress to overt hypothyroidism?

33%-55%

The risk of progression to overt hypothyroidism is associated with higher TSH levels (>12) and positive antithyroid peroxidase antibodies. True or false?

True

For patients with subclinical hypothyroidism, under what conditions may thyroid replacement treatment be considered?

- Symptomatic patients
- Patients with TSH >10, since treatment appears to prevent progression to overt hypothyroidism
- Pregnant patients with TSH >4.5, since subclinical hypothyroidism is a risk factor for miscarriage and low-birth weight
- Patients with goiters, since replacement can decrease goiter size

How do you treat hypothyroidism?	Synthetic L-thyroxine (T4) supplement
How do you measure response to hypothyroidism therapy?	Check TSH every 4-6 weeks until euthyroid (though symptoms can improve after 2 weeks)
How do you treat myxedema coma?	L-thyroxine IV

HYPERTHYROIDISM AND THYROTOXICOSIS

What is thyrotoxicosis?	A condition resulting from exposure of body tissues to excessive levels of thyroid hormones
What are the causes of thyrotoxicosis?	Hyperthyroidism, thyroiditis, exogenous thyroid intake

For the following systems, describe the clinical manifestations of thyrotoxicosis.

Dermatologic	Sweating, hair thinning, onycholysis (separation of nail from nail bed), warm skin
Cardiovascular	Tachycardia, wide pulse pressure, elevated systolic blood pressure, atrial fibrillation (in 10%-20% of patients with hyperthyroidism)
Respiratory	Increased oxygen consumption and respiratory muscle weakness leading to dyspnea
Gastrointestinal	Increased basal metabolic rate and increased gut motility leading to weight loss and diarrhea
Hematologic	Plasma volume increases more than RBC mass leading to normocytic anemia
Genitourinary	Urinary frequency, nocturia, anovulatory infertility, oligomenorrhea, amenorrhea
Musculoskeletal	Proximal muscle weakness, tremor (best seen in the outstretched hands or in the tongue), increased bone resorption leading to osteoporosis
Psychiatric	Anxiety

What is the single best lab test to assess thyroid function?

Thyroid-stimulating hormone (TSH)

Interpret these lab findings.

Elevated free T4 and low TSH

Thyrotoxicosis

Normal free T4 and low TSH

Subclinical hyperthyroidism

What test should you order if both free T4 and TSH are elevated?

MRI to look for a TSH-producing pituitary adenoma (can also present with a visual field defect)

Differentiate the causes of thyrotoxicosis based on thyroid size.

Diffusely enlarged goiter

Graves disease, toxic multinodular goiter (in countries with low iodine intake)

Palpable nodule

Thyroid adenoma

Normal

Subacute thyroiditis, exogenous hyperthyroidism (factitious vs. iatrogenic), ectopic hyperthyroidism (struma ovarii)

What is struma ovarii?

Functioning thyroid tissue in an ovarian neoplasm

What physical findings are unique to Graves disease?

Ophthalmopathy, infiltrative dermopathy

Describe the ophthalmopathy seen with Graves disease?

Stare, lid lag, exophthalmos

What is lid lag?

When a person with Graves disease looks down, the upper sclerae can be seen since the upper eyelid closes slowly.

What causes the exophthalmos in Graves disease?

The eye pushed outward secondary to inflammation of the extraocular muscles and orbital fat

Describe the infiltrative dermopathy seen with Graves disease.

Pretibial myxedema with raised, hyperpigmented, violaceous, orange-peel textured papules

Describe the pathology behind Graves disease?

An autoimmune disorder characterized by TSH receptor antibodies

Besides the physical examination, how can you diagnose the cause of thyrotoxicosis?	Radioactive iodine uptake (RAIU) scan
What does high radioiodine uptake indicate?	*De novo* hormone synthesis
Is treatment with radioiodine ablation or thionamides (methimazole and prophylthiouracil) appropriate?	Either will decrease hormone synthesis
What does low radioiodine uptake indicate?	Destruction of thyroid tissue with release of preformed hormone or an extrathyroidal source
Is treatment with radioiodine ablation or thionamides appropriate?	No
What are the causes of high radioiodine uptake?	Graves disease (uptake is diffuse), toxic adenoma, toxic multinodular goiter, TSH-producing pituitary adenoma, beta-human chorionic gonadotropin (hCG)-mediated hyperthyroidism
What are the causes of beta-hCG-mediated hyperthyroidism?	Hydatidiform mole, choriocarcinoma, testicular germ-cell cancer
Why does high beta-hCG cause hyperthyroidism?	Beta-hCG has some TSH-like activity due to their shared alpha subunit.
What are the causes of low radioiodine uptake?	Thyroiditis, exogenous thyroid ingestion, ectopic thyroid
What is thyroiditis?	Transient increase in thyroid hormones secondary to the release of preformed hormones
What are some causes of thyroiditis?	Viral/subacute, postpartum, chemical (amiodarone induced), post-radiation
How do you differentiate between the causes of subacute thyroiditis?	Subacute granulomatous thyroiditis is painful, while subacute lymphocytic thyroiditis is painless and often occurs postpartum (approximately 6 weeks postpartum).

How do you treat the beta-adrenergic symptoms (tachycardia, tremor) of thyrotoxicosis?	Propranolol
What are the main treatments of hyperthyroidism?	Thionamides, radioactive iodine ablation (ablation within 6-18 weeks), thyroidectomy
What supplementation will a patient need after undergoing ablation or surgery?	Levothyroxine
Which thionamide should be used during pregnancy?	Propylthiouracil (PTU), because it does not readily cross the placenta
What characteristics would make you more concerned that a thyroid nodule was malignant?	History of neck irradiation, "cold" nodule, male sex, firm and fixed solitary nodule
What is a "cold" nodule?	The absence of uptake in one nodular region on radioiodine uptake scan
What test should you order to evaluate a "cold" nodule?	Fine needle aspiration (FNA) of the nodule
How do you treat subacute thyroiditis?	Beta-blockers for thyrotoxicosis or levothyroxine for hypothyroidism, anti-inflammatory medications (eg, aspirin, ibuprofen, steroids)

CHAPTER 5

Osteoporosis

What percentage of postmenopausal women will have an osteoporosis-related fracture?	Approximately 50%
What are the risk factors for fractures *independent* of bone mineral density (BMD)?	Advanced age, previous fracture, long-term glucocorticoid therapy, body weight less than 127 pounds, first degree relative with a hip fracture, cigarette smoking, excessive alcohol intake
What is the preferred diagnostic modality for osteoporosis?	Bone mass density scan (DEXA) of the hip and lumbar spine
How is the T score calculated?	T score = (BMD [patient] − mean BMD [of a young adult population])/Standard deviation (of a young adult population)
What is a normal T score?	0 to −1
What T score defines osteopenia?	−1 to −2.5
Osteoporosis?	<−2.5
According to the US Preventive Services Task Force, who should be screened for osteoporosis?	Women aged 65 years and older, or younger women whose fracture risk is equal to or greater than that of a 65 year old white woman with no other risk factors.
How frequently should women be screened for osteoporosis?	The National Osteoporosis Foundation recommends screening every 2 years.
Men with what conditions should get a bone mass density test?	Low-trauma fractures, radiographic osteopenia, hypogonadism, irritable bowel disease, glucocorticoid therapy, primary hyperparathyroidism, loss of more than 1.5 in. in height

What are treatments for osteoporosis?	Bisphosphonates, selective estrogen receptor modulators (raloxifene), supplemental calcium and vitamin D, weight-bearing exercise (at least 30 minutes three times per week), smoking cessation
How much supplemental calcium?	1000 mg per day
How much supplemental vitamin D?	800 IU per day
What serum 25-hydroxyvitamin D (25OHD) concentration is defined as vitamin D insufficiency?	20-30 ng/mL
Vitamin D deficiency?	<20 ng/mL

What factors influence cutaneous production of vitamin D?

- Age: production declines with advancing age
- Latitude
- Cloud cover: complete cloud cover reduces UV energy by 50%
- Shade: shade and pollution decrease UV energy by 60%, UV energy does not penetrate glass
- Sunscreens: sun protection factors greater than 8 block vitamin D producing UV rays
- Skin melanin content: darker pigmentation is associated with less vitamin D production

Approximately how much sun exposure is needed to maintain an adequate amount of cutaneous vitamin D production?	Five to thirty minutes between 10 AM and 3 PM twice per week to the face, arms, legs, or back without sunscreen (varies by time of year and by latitude)
What is the treatment for vitamin D insufficiency?	800-1000 IU of oral vitamin D2 (ergocalciferol) or D3 (cholecalciferol) per day
What is the treatment for vitamin D deficiency?	50,000 IU of oral vitamin D2 or D3 once per week for 6-8 weeks, then 800-1000 IU of vitamin D2 or D3 daily (though the optimal dose and frequency are still being researched)
How do bisphosphonates work?	Bisphosphonates inhibit osteoclastic bone resorption.

How should bisphosphonates be taken?

On an empty stomach, first thing in the morning, with at least 8 ounces of water; nothing else by mouth for at least 30 minutes after ingestion; remain upright for at least 30 minutes after ingestion (to minimize esophageal side effects)

What is the risk of osteonecrosis of the jaw with oral bisphosphonate use?

1 in 100,000 patient years

Is hormone replacement therapy a first-line therapy for osteoporosis?

No. It is reserved for patients who have menopausal symptoms or cannot tolerate bisphosphonates.

Do bisphosphonates decrease fracture risk in patients with osteopenia?

No. Bisphosphonates have been shown to increase BMD in patients with osteopenia though this has not consistently led to fracture risk reduction.

What is the treatment of osteopenia?

Calcium and vitamin D, weight-bearing exercise, and smoking cessation. Bisphosphonates and selective estrogen receptor modulators are approved for the prevention of osteoporosis and can be considered in patients with increased fracture risk.

CHAPTER 6

Chronic Lung Disease

What are pulmonary function tests?

Pulmonary function testing (PFT) is a relatively simple battery of tests that quantify lung function in a reproducible manner. PFTs are used to diagnose and monitor a wide variety of pulmonary signs, symptoms and diseases.

What is the most widely used component of pulmonary function testing?

Spirometry

What is forced expiratory volume in one second (FEV$_1$)?

It is a dynamic spirometric test which evaluates the mechanical properties of the large- and medium-sized airways. FEV$_1$ is a measure of the air volume a person forcefully expires in the first second of expiration following maximal inspiration.

What is forced vital capacity (FVC)?

It is a static spirometric test measuring the total air volume a person can expire after inhaling maximally.

How is FVC related to total lung capacity?

Decreased FVC is usually due to reduced lung capacity (in a restrictive process). However, FVC is *not* equivalent or even necessarily proportional to total lung capacity. Reduced airflow, air trapping, and/or increased residual volume decrease FVC in obstructive processes.

How are the normal FEV$_1$ and FVC reference values established?

Normal values are based on population studies according to gender, age, height, and race. Patient's FEV$_1$ and FVC can be expressed as either absolute numbers or as a percent predicted of normal (patient's value divided by average population value).

What *percent of predicted* is considered normal FEV$_1$ and FVC?

80%-100%

FEV$_1$ normally equals about what percent of FVC?

The normal FEV$_1$/FVC ratio changes with age

Age (in years)	FEV$_1$/FVC
8-19	85%
20-39	80%
40-59	75%
60-80	70%

Are FEV$_1$, FVC, FEV$_1$/FVC low, high, or normal in obstructive versus restrictive lung diseases? What characterizes these diseases?

	FEV$_1$	FVC	FEV$_1$/FVC	Lung Characteristics
Obstructive	Low	Low or normal	Low	Air trapping Increased volume Airflow restriction Normal or increased compliance
Restrictive	Low or normal	Low	Normal or high	Reduced volume Reduced compliance

Why do some restrictive diseases have a normal or high FEV$_1$/FVC?

Both FEV$_1$ and FVC are low. If they are proportionately low, the FEV$_1$/FVC ratio is normal. If FVC is disproportionately low, the ratio is high.

What are the two most common obstructive lung diseases?

Asthma and chronic obstructive pulmonary disease (COPD)

Do the following conditions cause obstructive or restrictive pulmonary disease?

Kyphosis	Restrictive
Idiopathic pulmonary fibrosis	Restrictive
Cystic fibrosis	Obstructive
Asbestosis	Restrictive
Sarcoidosis	Restrictive
Bronchiectasis	Obstructive
Berylliosis	Restrictive
Beryllium disease	Restrictive
Neuromuscular disease	Restrictive

What genetic (autosomal recessive) disease causes pancreatic insufficiency and frequent pulmonary infections secondary to mucus plugs?

Cystic fibrosis

What is bronchiectasis?

Permanent dilation and destruction of bronchi usually caused by frequent severe infections and/or inflammation

ASTHMA

What is the most common chronic lung disease in children?

Asthma

What is asthma?

A chronic lung disease in which smooth muscle contraction, airway wall thickening (edema, vasodilation, inflammatory cell infiltrates), and intraluminal debris and mucus cause episodes of airway obstruction

Does asthma worsen over time?

Asthma is *usually* not a progressive disease. However, patients may experience periods of exacerbations and remissions.

In some patients, what lung structure changes occur over time and progressively reduce airway obstruction reversibility?

Thickening of sub-basement membrane, subepithelial fibrosis, airway smooth muscle hypertrophy, angiogenesis, mucus gland hyperplasia

Clinical studies should include spirometry at the time of diagnosis (and subsequently for monitoring purposes) in all patients starting at what age?

Most children are developmentally ready at 5 years.

In most asthma patients, how is airway obstruction evident when measuring FEV_1 before bronchodilator therapy?

Asthma is a disease of airway obstruction and therefore, FEV_1 is usually reduced in the absence of a bronchodilator.

In most asthma patients, how is airway obstruction reversibility evident when measuring FEV_1 post-bronchodilator therapy?

Post-bronchodilator FEV_1 improvement indicates reversibility. Reversibility is more common in asthma than COPD. Reversibility is defined by a FEV_1 post-bronchodilator improvement of 12% and 200 mL. Larger changes become less likely to be COPD and more likely to be asthma.

Occasionally patients with severe untreated asthma may not show obstruction reversibility with a bronchodilator. What strategy is used in this scenario?

The patient may require 2-3 weeks of oral glucocorticoid therapy prior to the test to demonstrate reversibility.

If a patient with suspected asthma has normal (or near-normal) spirometry measurements, a bronchial provocation can help establish the diagnosis. Describe this test.

It is an inhalation challenge test used in the PFT laboratory. The patient is exposed to stages of progressively increasing concentrations of methacholine (although challenge can also be done with histamine, cold air, or exercise). The patient performs spirometry at each stage.

What constitutes a positive versus negative bronchial provocation?

A 20% FEV_1 reduction in response to the provocation is a positive test for airway hyperresponsiveness. The test is negative if the FEV_1 drops less than 20% through the entire test.

A positive bronchial provocation test establishes the diagnosis of asthma. True or false?

False. It strongly suggests a diagnosis of asthma, but there are other diseases that produce a positive result. However, a negative test reliably excludes the diagnosis of asthma.

During a diagnostic workup, what value do a CXR and EKG provide?

Patients usually have a normal CXR and EKG. These tests should not be done routinely but are useful in excluding pulmonary and cardiac conditions suspected of mimicking or compounding asthma symptoms.

What is Samter triad?

1. Asthma
2. Nasal polyps
3. Aspirin sensitivity

What is the atopic triad (chronic conditions associated with asthma)?

1. Asthma
2. Atopic dermatitis (eczema)
3. Allergic rhinitis

What are some examples of common asthma triggers?

Exercise, upper respiratory infection, allergens, irritants, cold/dry weather, gastroesophageal reflux disease, and physical or emotional stress

When is allergy testing beneficial?

Many asthma patients having notable allergies and knowledge obtained from allergy testing may aid in avoiding these asthma triggers.

What are the three main symptoms of asthma?

1. End expiratory wheezing
2. Dyspnea/Chest tightness
3. Cough

Besides asthma, what are some other causes of wheezing in children?

Anything that restricts the airways: infection (bronchiolitis, pneumonia, etc), foreign body aspiration, congenital heart disease, tracheomalacia, cystic fibrosis

In some patients, coughing may be the only symptom of asthma. True or false?

True. This occurs more often in children than adults. Coughing usually occurs at night or is associated with exercise. A positive response to asthma medication confirms the diagnosis.

Based on symptom frequency, what are the four classifications of asthma?

Mild intermittent (<2 symptoms per week), mild persistent (>2 symptoms per week), moderate persistent (daily symptoms), severe persistent (continuous symptoms)

Regardless of classification, an adequate prophylactic medication regimen should reduce the frequency of breakthrough asthma symptoms to how many times per week?

<2

What is the preferred class of medications for treatment of breakthrough symptoms that occur despite prophylactic measures?

Inhaled short-acting beta-2 agonists (SABA), known as "rescue inhalers," such as albuterol

What is more efficacious, a SABA administered by inhaler or nebulizer?

If used correctly, they are equally efficacious. People using inhalers may find spacers helpful. Young children usually need a nebulizer for proper delivery of medication.

What class of medication is used to treat mild intermittent asthma?

Because symptoms occur twice a week or less, a patient with mild intermittent asthma only needs a SABA to use as needed.

Inhaled glucocorticosteroids are the mainstay of pharmacologic asthma therapy and should be prescribed as first-line prophylaxis for most patients experiencing symptoms more than twice weekly. True or false?

True. Inflammation is a central feature of asthma.

What are alternative first-line medications?

Cromolyn, leukotriene receptor antagonist (LTRA), nedocromil, or theophylline

Which one is rarely used because it has a narrow therapeutic index and requires monitoring of levels to avoid toxicity?

Theophylline

Which ones work as mast cell stabilizers (inhibit histamine release)?

Cromolyn, nedocromil

Montelukast and zafirlukast are examples of which medication class?

Leukotriene receptor antagonists

When a low-dose inhaled steroid (or alternative first-line medication) fails to manage asthma symptoms adequately, what are the options for treatment management?

Increase dose of inhaled steroid; use inhaled steroid *plus* one of the following: inhaled long-acting beta-2 agonist (LABA), LTRA, theophylline, or zileuton; and/or add oral steroids (severe cases). Refer to pulmonologist or immunologist as needed.

According to the US Food and Drug Administration, what risks are associated with taking a LABA as single-agent therapy?

LABAs taken alone can decrease the frequency of asthma attacks but increase the severity of those attacks when they do occur; they may also disguise uncontrolled asthma. LABAs should be taken in conjunction with a steroid and only when the steroid is not adequately controlling symptoms. Some inhalers combine a LABA and steroid for easier administration.

What is zileuton and what precautions should be taken with its use?

It is an oral medication that inhibits leukotriene formation. There are limited studies on this medication compared to alternative therapies. It may cause liver toxicity and thus requires close lab monitoring.

What is the treatment for exercise-induced asthma?

The treatment of choice is a SABA 15-30 minutes prior to exercise. Cromolyn is an alternative. LABAs are helpful in some situations (eg, schoolchild can take it in the morning and effects last through an afternoon sports activity) but are safe only if the patient is also on a steroid.

What device can patients use to quantitatively self-assess their lung function (in an acute exacerbation or to gauge prophylactic medication effectiveness)?

Peak expiratory flow rate (PEFR) monitor

What is an asthma action plan?

A written plan established by the patient and doctor which describes the patient's asthma triggers, normal and abnormal peak flow ranges, asthma symptoms (mild to moderate versus severe), medication protocols, and emergency instructions

What is status asthmaticus?

A life-threatening asthma attack that is unresponsive to standard inhaled medication (bronchodilators and steroids) and requires emergency care

Can anybody with asthma have a severe asthma attack?

Yes. Although patients with undertreated disease or severe underlying disease are generally more likely to have severe attacks, even patients with mild asthma have the potential for a life-threatening event.

What physical signs may indicate a severe asthma exacerbation?

Peak flow rate less than 50% of predicted normal, severe wheezing or cessation of audible wheezing (air flow is so diminished that wheezing can no longer be appreciated), tachypnea, severe retraction and nasal flaring, breathlessness not relieved by rescue inhaler, tachycardia, cyanosis, diaphoresis

What is the treatment of a severe asthma exacerbation?

Frequent or continuous inhaled beta-2 agonist, oral or intravenous corticosteroids, subcutaneous or intramuscular epinephrine, and/or oxygen supplementation or mechanical ventilation

Why is an elevated $PaCO_2$ of particular concern during a severe asthma attack?

Patients typically hyperventilate during an attack and thus have a low $PaCO_2$. An elevated $PaCO_2$ may indicate patient fatigue and impending respiratory failure.

COPD

What is COPD?

A chronic lung disease characterized by airflow limitation caused by airway disease (inflammation, increased mucus) and parenchymal destruction

What is the strongest risk factor associated with the development of COPD?

Smoking

Does COPD worsen over time?

Yes. Unlike asthma, COPD tends to be a progressive disease, especially if exposure to harmful substances (usually smoking) continues. Reduction or elimination of exposures can significantly reduce the rate of lung function deterioration.

What are the two types of COPD?

Chronic bronchitis and emphysema

What is chronic bronchitis?

A chronic expiratory airflow obstruction with cough and excessive sputum production for at least 3 months in a year for 2 years

What is emphysema?

Chronic expiratory airflow obstruction with enlargement of the airspaces, destruction of alveoli, and loss of elasticity of alveolar walls

Panacinar emphysema and liver cirrhosis developing in a young non-smoking patient is most likely due to what genetic disease?

Alpha 1-antitrypsin deficiency

What are the common symptoms associated with COPD?

Cough, dyspnea, excessive sputum production

Patients with COPD have what typical findings on chest x-ray?

Usually normal, but in *advanced* disease you may see flattened diaphragms, enlarged lung fields, increased AP diameter, or interstitial markings with bullae

Patients with COPD have what typical findings on EKG?

Usually normal, but you may see poor R-wave progression in leads V1-V6, right-sided heart strain, or low-voltage QRS due to increased chest diameter

Do you have to document airflow obstruction on PFTs to make the diagnosis of COPD?

Yes. COPD is not a clinical diagnosis but one that is made by spirometry.

In COPD, is residual lung volume increased or decreased compared to patients without COPD?

Increased

In most COPD patients, what do spirometric measurements (FEV_1, FEV_1/FVC) show pre- and post-bronchodilator therapy?

Reduced FEV_1 pre-bronchodilator therapy indicates airway obstruction. Airway obstruction is largely irreversible, some COPD patients show mild post-bronchodilator FEV_1 improvements, especially if their disease has a component of asthma. However, the post-bronchodilator FEV_1/FVC ratio always remains below 0.7 in COPD.

The Global Initiative for Chronic Obstructive Pulmonary Disease (GOLD) recommends taking diagnostic spirometric measurements after administration of a bronchodilator to reduce testing variability. According to GOLD, what FEV_1/FVC and FEV_1 values are consistent with COPD?

In COPD, post-bronchodilator FEV_1/FVC is less than 0.7 and FEV_1 is less than 80% of predicted.

According to GOLD, how are the stages of COPD defined?

Mild (Stage I)

FEV/FVC <70%, FEV_1 ≥80% predicted, with or without symptoms

Moderate (Stage II)

FEV_1/FVC <70%, FEV_1 = 50%-80% predicted, dyspnea with exertion, without or without cough and sputum production

Severe (Stage III)

FEV_1/FVC <70%, FEV_1 = 30%-50% predicted, increased dyspnea, reduced exercise capacity, fatigue, repeated exacerbations

Very severe (Stage IV)

FEV_1/FVC <70%, FEV_1 <30% predicted, or FEV_1 <50% plus respiratory failure

Inhaled glucocorticosteroids are the mainstay of pharmacologic COPD therapy and should be prescribed as first-line treatment for most patients. True or false?

False. Bronchodilators are central to symptomatic management of COPD.

According to the GOLD, what is the treatment for each COPD stage?

Mild (Stage I)

Short-acting bronchodilator when needed

Moderate (Stage II)

Treatment for Stage I, one or more daily long-acting beta-agonists or anticholinergics, pulmonary rehabilitation

Severe (Stage III)

Treatment for Stage II, inhaled glucocorticosteroids for repeated exacerbations

Very severe (Stage IV)

Treatment for Stage III, long-term oxygen therapy if indicated, consider surgical treatments

What are the different classes of bronchodilators used in the treatment of COPD?

Anticholinergics (eg, ipratropium), short- and long-acting beta-agonists, methylxanthines (eg, theophylline)

Salmeterol is an example of what type of bronchodilator?

Long-acting beta-2 agonist

How do anticholinergics help keep airways open?

They inhibit muscarinic cholinergic receptors and reduce intrinsic vagal tone of airways.

Do steroids slow the FEV_1 decline of COPD?

No

What is the benefit of corticosteroids in a COPD patient?

They decrease exacerbations and are useful in an acute setting.

What are the only interventions that have consistently shown effectiveness in decreasing *mortality* due to COPD?

Smoking cessation decreases the progression of lung damage due to COPD, no matter how early or advanced the disease. Oxygen prolongs life in patients with oxygen insufficiency.

What interventions improve *morbidity* in COPD patients?

Medications, smoking cessation, oxygen therapy, influenza and pneumococcal vaccines, pulmonary rehabilitation

What are the components of pulmonary rehabilitation?

Exercise conditioning, breathing retraining, education, psychological support

In what ways does pulmonary rehabilitation improve morbidity due to COPD?

It enhances quality of life by reducing anxiety and depression symptoms, reducing hospitalization rates, and improving exercise performance. It does *not* improve overall pulmonary function.

What are the indications for *continuous* long-term home oxygen therapy in patients with COPD?

1. Arterial PO_2 ≤55 mm Hg or oxygen saturation ≤88%

or

2. Arterial PO_2 from 55-59 mm Hg or oxygen saturation ≤89% PLUS one of the following:
   - Dependent edema secondary to congestive heart failure
   - Evidence of cor pulmonale
   - Evidence of pulmonary hypertension
   - Erythrocytosis (hematocrit >56%)

The chronic course of COPD is punctuated by acute exacerbations. Answer the following questions regarding acute exacerbations of COPD.

What is the most common cause?	Infection (viruses, *Streptococcus pneumoniae* and *Moraxella catarrhalis*)
What are other causes?	Cardiac failure or arrhythmias, chest trauma, pneumothorax, pulmonary embolism, iatrogenic (inappropriate doses of beta-blockers, narcotics, etc)
What are the symptoms?	Worsening dyspnea, chest tightness, and cough; wheezing; increased sputum production/tenacity
What physical signs indicate a severe exacerbation?	Use of accessory muscles and paradoxical chest movement, cyanosis, signs of heart failure (eg, edema, hemodynamic instability), mental status changes
What conditions can mimic an exacerbation?	Infection (pneumonia), pulmonary embolism, pneumothorax, pleural effusion, cardiac condition (arrhythmia, heart failure)
What is the workup of COPD exacerbations?	Arterial blood gases, CXR, EKG, labs (CBC, BMP, BNP), spiral CT if pulmonary embolism is suspected
What is the treatment?	Bronchodilator therapy, oxygen (keep O_2 saturation at 90%-94%), oral or IV corticosteroids, antibiotics for exacerbations caused by bacterial infections
Why should you monitor PCO_2 while on O_2 therapy?	Oxygen can decrease the respiratory drive, causing the individual's PCO_2 to increase
What is the treatment of hypercapnia?	BiPAP followed by intubation if needed
What does "BiPAP" stand for?	Bi-level (variable) positive airway pressure
What does BiPAP do?	Mechanically delivers air through a mask at one pressure for inhaling (high) and at another for exhaling (low)

In COPD patients, what are the most common causes of pneumonia?

Viruses, *H. influenzae, S. pneumoniae, M. catarrhalis*

What is cor pulmonale?

Cor pulmonale is right-sided heart failure resulting from long-term increased pressure in the pulmonary vasculature and right ventricle. It can be caused by a number of chronic pulmonary conditions, including COPD.

CHAPTER 7

Attention Deficit and Hyperactivity Disorder (ADHD)

What percentage of the population has been diagnosed with ADHD?	5%
ADHD symptoms can be grouped into which 3 categories?	Hyperactivity, impulsivity, inattention
Describe the following ADHD symptoms.	
Hyperactivity	Excessive fidgetiness or talking, difficulty playing quietly, frequent restlessness, difficulty remaining seated
Impulsivity	Blurting out answers too quickly, difficulty waiting turns, interrupting others' activities
Inattention	Forgetfulness, losing or misplacing things, disorganization, poor attention to detail, being easily distracted, avoiding tasks that require sustained mental efforts

Answer the following questions about ADHD with respect to the *Diagnostic and Statistical Manual of Mental Disorders (DSM)-IV* criteria.

Symptoms of inattention or hyperactivity-impulsivity should persist for how long?

At least 6 months

Impairment should be present before which age?

Before 7 years of age

Impairment should occur in how many settings?

In 2 or more settings (social, academic, occupational)

What conditions should be excluded?

Other mental disorders that could account for the symptoms

In evaluating a patient with ADHD symptoms, what other conditions should be considered?

Learning disabilities, intellectual disability, depression, bipolar disease, anxiety, post-traumatic stress disorder, conduct disorder, oppositional defiant disorder, substance abuse, stressful home environment, lead poisoning, hearing/visual impairment, asthma, fetal alcohol syndrome, thyroid abnormalities, sleep disorders, seizure disorders

Are the following statements true or false?

According to the American Academy of Pediatrics, obtaining information regarding symptoms (functional impairment, age of onset, duration) exclusively from the patient's parents is sufficient to make a diagnosis of ADHD.

False. Information from parents (or caregivers) *and* teachers is needed to make the diagnosis.

Routine diagnostic tests such as lead levels, thyroid tests, and EEGs are indicated to establish the diagnosis of ADHD.

False. These tests are not routine but can be used as deemed necessary (based on history and physical) to assess the existence of coexisting conditions.

What percentage of children with ADHD have one or more comorbid conditions such as oppositional defiant disorder, conduct disorder, and depression?

50%

What medications can be used to treat ADHD?

Stimulants (eg, methylphenidate, dextroamphetamine, and mixed amphetamine salts), atomoxetine, tricyclic antidepressants, bupropion, clonidine

A positive response to a trial of stimulants confirms the diagnosis of ADHD. True or false?

False. Children with learning disabilities and depression will also respond to stimulants.

What side effects are associated with stimulants?

Anorexia (80%), sleep disturbances (up to 85%), tics (15%-30%), weight loss (10%-15%), mania, increased heart rate, increased blood pressure, nervousness, mania, deceleration of linear growth (though adult height is not affected)

Tourette syndrome is an absolute contraindication for stimulant therapy in patients with ADHD. True or false?

False. Children with Tourette syndrome and ADHD can benefit from certain doses of stimulants without the worsening of tics.

Do stimulants increase the risk of sudden cardiac death in patients without known cardiac disease?

No studies have established a causal relationship. However, the Food and Drug Administration recommended that stimulants carry a warning after there were reports of sudden unexpected death in children on stimulants.

What is the AAP recommendation regarding routine electrocardiograms before initiating stimulant therapy?

An EKG is not needed before initiating stimulant therapy, unless the child is known to have cardiac disease or the history or physical exam is suggestive of cardiac disease.

What medication should be used in patients with ADHD and illicit substance abuse?

Atomoxetine (a selective norepinephrine reuptake inhibitor) is an acceptable alternative to stimulants and should be considered in patients that are not candidates for stimulant therapy.

What percentage of children with ADHD will continue to have symptoms into adult life?

30%-70%

Diagnosing ADHD in adult patients requires that he/she meet *DSM-IV* criteria. True or false?

True. The provider should inquire about academic grades, conduct in school, and psychiatric history and should consider obtaining evidence (with patient consent) from a patient's employer, spouse, and co-workers.

CHAPTER 8

Depression and Anxiety

DEPRESSION

What age group has the highest incidence of depression?	25-34 years
What age group is twice as likely to commit suicide as the general population?	Elderly
What diseases can present with depressive symptoms?	Thyroid problems, Parkinson disease, viral illnesses, carcinoid syndrome, cancer (especially pancreatic cancer), systemic lupus erythematosus (SLE), cerebrovascular disease
What are some common medications/ substances that can induce depression?	Alcohol, beta-blockers, barbiturates, steroids, anticonvulsants, diuretics, stimulant withdrawal
What are the symptoms of major depression?	SIGECAPS:

SIGECAPS:

Decreased **S**leep (early morning awakenings common)

Loss of **I**nterest

Feelings of **G**uilt

Loss of **E**nergy

Decreased **C**oncentration

Change in **A**ppetite

Change in **P**sychomotor activity

Suicidal ideation

How long must a person have a depressed mood (or anhedonia) in addition to at least four of the above symptoms in order to have a diagnosis of a major depressive episode?	Two weeks
Episodic depression occurring only during months with fewer daylight hours, and often characterized by irritability, hypersomnia, and carbohydrate craving is what subtype of major depressive disorders?	Seasonal affective disorder
What is the nonpharmacologic therapy for seasonal affective disorder?	Light therapy
What are the most common side effects of selective serotonin reuptake inhibitors (SSRIs)?	Headache, gastrointestinal (GI) complaints, sexual dysfunction
What are the most common side effects of tricyclic antidepressants (TCAs)?	Sedation, weight gain, orthostatic hypotension, anticholinergic side effects (dry mouth, dizziness, urinary retention, constipation), prolonged QT syndrome
A patient who is on a monoamine oxidase inhibitor (MAOI) runs out of medications so she borrows her friend's antidepressant medication (SSRI). Later, she presents to the emergency department with autonomic instability, hyperthermia, and seizures. What is the diagnosis?	Serotonin syndrome
A patient who presents 3 months after the loss of a loved one with feeling of guilt, mild sleep disturbance, visual or auditory hallucinations of the deceased person, and weight loss is most likely experiencing what reaction?	Normal grief (bereavement)
If the above symptoms persisted for more than a year, or involved suicidal ideation, what would be your diagnosis?	Abnormal grief (major depression)
Why is it important to screen a patient for manic symptoms before starting a patient on an antidepressant?	Antidepressants such as SSRIs can trigger a manic episode in bipolar disorder.

What are the symptoms of a manic episode?

DIG FAST:

Distractibility

Insomnia

Grandiosity

Flight of ideas

Increased goal-directed **A**ctivity

Pressured **S**peech

Thoughts racing

What is the pharmacologic treatment of Bipolar I/II disorders?

Anticonvulsants (eg, carbamazepine, valproic acid), lithium, atypical antipsychotics (eg, olanzapine, aripiprazole, risperidone)

How does depression manifest itself differently in children as opposed to adults?

Children often present with irritability instead of depressed mood

What percentage of new mothers experience postpartum depression?

10%

What emergent side effect of trazodone must you warn patients about?

Priapism

What does a person taking an MAOI need to avoid?

Tyramine-rich foods (cheese and wine), pseudoephedrine (hypertensive crisis), TCAs (hyperpyrexia), meperidine (serotonin syndrome), SSRIs (serotonin syndrome)

What antidepressant is classically associated with an increased incidence of seizures?

Bupropion

What class of drugs is associated with cardiac dysrhythmias and can be lethal in overdose?

TCAs (limit quantities of these drugs in potentially suicidal patients)

Why do physicians need to closely monitor a child on an antidepressant?

Antidepressant use is associated with an increased risk of suicidal ideation and suicide-related behaviors in children

What are the indications for electroconvulsive therapy (ECT)?

Unresponsiveness to pharmacotherapy, intolerable side effects of pharmacotherapy (elderly), need for rapid symptom decrease (high suicidality)

What is the major side effect of ECT?	Retrograde amnesia
What percent of patients with eating disorders also have depression?	50%-75%
What eating disorder is characterized by a fear of and refusal to gain weight despite weighing less than 85% of expected?	Anorexia nervosa
What eating disorder is characterized by a lack of control over eating followed by compensatory behavior to gain weight (self-induced vomiting, misuse of medications such as laxatives, excessive exercise, fasting)?	Bulimia nervosa

ANXIETY DISORDERS

What is the lifetime prevalence of anxiety disorders?	30% in women and 19% in men
A patient who describes himself as a "chronic worrier" and has had persistent, hard to control anxiety for more than 6 months, along with insomnia and fatigue most likely has what diagnosis?	Generalized anxiety disorder (GAD)
What is the treatment for GAD?	Buspirone (or other azaspirones), SSRI, or serotonin-norepinephrine reuptake inhibitor (venlafaxine, duloxetine), all in combination with psychotherapy. Benzodiazepines are acceptable for acute anxiety, but not ideal for long-term management.
Recurrent episodes of palpitations, GI distress, dyspnea, and feelings of impending doom that last 5-10 minutes are typical of what disorder?	Panic disorder
What conditions should be ruled out before treatment of suspected panic attacks?	Angina, myocardial infarction, side effects of sympathomimetic drugs, thyrotoxicosis, carcinoid syndrome, pheochromocytoma, pulmonary embolism

Is panic disorder more common in men or women?

Twice as common in women than men

What drugs are considered first-line treatment to prevent panic attacks from recurring?

SSRIs. Benzodiazepines can be added to treat disabling symptoms

If a patient with panic disorder also relays to you that she has stopped going to the grocery store, prefers to shop online as opposed to at the mall, and no longer likes riding in elevators, what is your diagnosis?

Panic disorder with agoraphobia

What type of non-pharmacologic therapy is often recommended as an adjunct for the treatment of phobias?

Cognitive behavioral therapy (CBT)

Strong, exaggerated, and irrational fears of things such as animals, heights, or air travel, are known as what types of phobias?

Specific phobias

What is the nonpharmacologic treatment for phobias?

Systematic desensitization and supportive psychotherapy

Irrational fears of situations that can be embarrassing, such as public speaking, making small talk at parties, or using public restrooms, are known as what type of phobias?

Social phobias (social anxiety disorder)

What is the only medication approved for the treatment of social phobias?

Paroxetine is the only Food and Drug Administration (FDA)-approved SSRI.

A young female is distressed because she has had persistent thoughts that she has left her front door unlocked at night and gets up multiple times at night to check if it is locked. She knows this is "crazy," and is so sleep-deprived that she has been falling asleep. What disorder do you suspect?

Obsessive-compulsive disorder (OCD)

What is the difference between OCD and obsessive-compulsive personality disorder (OCPD)?

People with OCD have obsessions and compulsions that cause distress and prompt them to seek medical help. The actions of people with OCPD may cause relationship conflicts but do not cause a personal sense of distress. OCD symptoms fluctuate, but OCDP is chronic.

What are the first-line medications for OCD?

SSRIs or TCAs

What nonpharmacologic therapy can also be utilized as an adjunct to pharmacotherapy in a patient with OCD?

Exposure and response prevention

SECTION II

Common Chief Complaints

CHAPTER 9

Headache

90% of headaches fall under which three headache diagnoses?	Migraines, tension headaches, cluster headaches
What signs and symptoms suggest that the headache has a secondary cause and is not a migraine, tension headache, or cluster headache?	Sudden onset, onset after the age of 50, increasing frequency or severity, headache with concomitant systemic illness, focal neurologic signs, papilledema, trauma, headaches at night or early morning

The following signs and symptoms are associated with which secondary headache diagnoses?

New onset of headaches in patients 50 years of age or older	Temporal arteritis, intracranial mass
Sudden onset of severe headache (worst headache of the patient's life)	Subarachnoid hemorrhage
Headache with signs of systemic illness (fever, stiff neck, rash)	Meningitis, encephalitis, Lyme disease
Focal neurologic signs or symptoms	Intracranial mass, arteriovenous malformation, stroke
Papilledema	Intracranial mass, pseudotumor cerebri, meningitis
History of cancer	Intracranial metastases
History of HIV	Opportunistic infection (eg, cryptococcus, toxoplasmosis, tuberculosis, herpes), aseptic meningitis, intracranial mass (eg, lymphoma), progressive multifocal leukoencephalopathy
Headache during pregnancy or postpartum	Preeclampsia, venous sinus thrombosis, dissection, pituitary apoplexy
Chronic nasal congestion	Sinusitis
Headache after trauma	Subdural hemorrhage, epidural hemorrhage, posttraumatic headache
Headache in the temples associated with clicking or locking of the jaw	Temporomandibular joint (TMJ) disorder

MIGRAINES

What patient populations are most prone to migraine headaches?	Women, aged 30-39 years, positive family history for migraines
What are the types of migraines?	Migraines with aura, migraines without aura, migraine variants (including retinal, ophthalmoplegic, and familial hemiplegic migraines)
Which type is most common?	Migraine without aura (80%)
What are the International Headache Society diagnostic criteria for migraine headaches?	The headache must meet these three criteria: 1. Last between 4 and 72 hours 2. Have two of the following characteristics: unilateral, pulsating, aggravated by physical activity, moderate to severe in intensity 3. Be associated with one of the following symptoms: nausea/vomiting, photophobia/phonophobia
What are examples of auras?	Auras are typically reversible and can include visual (flickering lights, spots, lines, loss of vision), sensory (pins, needles, numbness), and speech symptoms.
What factors can trigger migraines?	Stress, menstruation, visual stimuli, weather changes, nitrates, fasting, wine, sleep disturbances, aspartame
What will migraine sufferers typically do to decrease symptoms?	Lie down in a quiet, dark room
What is the purpose of a headache diary?	A diary helps identify headache precipitating factors. These factors may be avoidable altogether, or patients may be able to time the use of prophylactic medications more appropriately (eg, just before menses).
What are pharmacologic treatment options for migraine headaches?	• Mild analgesics: ibuprofen, naproxen, diclofenac, aspirin, indomethacin, and acetaminophen • Triptans: sumatriptan, zolmitriptan • Ergots: ergotamine, dihydroergotamine • Antiemetics: metoclopramide • Dexamethasone

When should triptans be avoided?

Familial hemiplegic migraine, basilar migraine, ischemic stroke, ischemic heart disease, Prinzmetal angina, uncontrolled hypertension, pregnancy, monoamine oxidase inhibitor use, ergot use over the last 24 hours

What is the role of opioids in migraine treatment?

They should be reserved for patients with intractable migraines who are not responding to other abortive treatments. Routine use can be habit forming and contribute to rebound headaches.

What are the indications for preventive migraine therapy?

Frequent headaches (more than four per month); long-lasting headaches (>12 hours); headaches that cause significant disability; contraindications, refractory symptoms, or adverse events with acute medications

What medications can be used to prevent migraines?

- Beta-blockers: propranolol, metoprolol, atenolol
- Calcium channel blockers: verapamil, nifedipine
- ACE inhibitors/angiotension receptor blockers: lisinopril, candesartan
- Antidepressants: amitriptyline, nortriptyline, mirtazapine
- Anticonvulsants: valproate, gabapentin, topiramate

CLUSTER HEADACHES

How common are cluster headaches?

Affect <1% of the population and mostly affect males

What are the International Headache Society diagnostic criteria for cluster headaches?

1. Severe unilateral orbital, supraorbital, and/or temporal pain lasting 15-180 minutes
2. Be associated with one of the following ipsilateral signs: conjunctival injection, lacrimation, nasal congestion, rhinorrhea, facial sweating, miosis, ptosis, eyelid edema

Why are they called cluster headaches?

These headaches present in clusters, with up to eight episodes per day, followed by spontaneous periods of remission lasting days to months to years between attacks.

How are cluster headaches classified?

They can be classified as episodic or chronic depending on the extent of pain-free remissions between cycles. The chronic state is defined as cluster headaches occurring everyday for more than one year without a remission period lasting more than 1 month.

In general, patients with cluster headaches are like migraine sufferers in that they prefer to be in a dark quiet room when they have a headache. True or false?

False, patients with cluster headaches are restless and prefer to pace.

What are first line acute treatments for cluster headaches?

Oxygen (typically administered using a non-rebreathing facial mask with a flow rate of at least 7 L/min for 20 minutes) and triptans (subcutaneous or intranasal sumatriptan, oral or intranasal zolmitriptan)

What are second line acute treatments for cluster headaches?

Oral ergotamine, IV dihydroergotamine, intranasal lidocaine, subcutaneous octreotide

When should preventive medication be started for cluster headaches?

Start at the onset of a cluster episode and continue over the expected duration of the cluster period

Which preventive medications can be used for cluster headaches?

Verapamil, glucocorticoids, lithium, topiramate, methysergide

TENSION HEADACHES

What are the International Headache Society diagnostic criteria for tension headaches?

1. At least two of the following pain characteristics: pressing or tightening (nonpulsating) quality, mild or moderate intensity, bilateral location, no aggravation with routine physical activity
2. Not associated with nausea/vomiting or photophobia/phonophobia

What factors can trigger tension headaches?

Stress, certain head and neck movements

What abortive medications can be used to treat tension headaches?

Nonsteroidal anti-inflammatories (ibuprofen, naproxen, ketorolac), acetaminophen, combined acetaminophen or aspirin with caffeine, heat, ice, massage

DRUG REBOUND HEADACHES

When would you consider the diagnosis of drug rebound headache?

Routine ingestion of medications for headache (approximately three times per week), symptoms are refractory to acute and prophylactic interventions

Which medications can cause drug rebound headaches?

Any acute headache medication can cause these headaches (acetaminophen, butalbital-aspirin-caffeine, aspirin, ergots, opioids, and triptans).

What is the management for drug rebound headaches?

- Stop all chronically used acute headache medications
- Use transitional agents during detoxification: intranasal/intramuscular dihydroergotamine, long acting triptans (naratriptan or frovatriptan), a short course of steroids, or long-acting NSAIDs
- Initiation of preventive medications

INTRACRANIAL HEMORRHAGE

What are the four major types of intracranial hemorrhage?

Epidural hematoma, subdural hematoma, subarachnoid hemorrhage, intracerebral hemorrhage

What causes an epidural hematoma?

Bleeding from meningeal arteries (classically, the middle meningeal artery)

What percent of epidural hematomas are associated with a skull fracture?

85%

How do you recognize an epidural hematoma?

The classic history describes head trauma with loss of consciousness, followed by a lucid interval, and then immediate neurologic deterioration.

What causes a subdural hematoma?

Bleeding from bridging veins between the cortex and venous sinuses

What patient populations are vulnerable to subdural hematomas?

Elderly and alcoholics

How do you differentiate between an epidural hematoma and subdural hematoma on CT scan?

An epidural hematoma is lenticular or biconvex in shape, while a subdural hematoma is crescent-shaped.

What causes a subarachnoid hemorrhage?

Bleeding between the arachnoid and pia mater, usually secondary to trauma or a berry aneurysm rupture

How do you make a definitive diagnosis of a subarachnoid hemorrhage?

A lumbar puncture demonstrates blood or xanthochromia. A CT may or may not show blood in the ventricles and surrounding brain and brainstem.

MENINGITIS

What are the most common bacterial meningitis pathogens in the following age groups.

<1 month?

Group B Streptococcus > Gram negative bacilli > Streptococcus pneumoniae

1 to 3 months?

Group B Streptococcus > Escherichia coli > Listeria monocytogenes

3 months to 3 years?

Streptococcus pneumoniae > Neisseria meningitidis > Group B streptococcus

3 years to 10 years?

Streptococcus pneumoniae > Neisseria meningitidis

10 years to 19 years?

Neisseria meningitidis

Adults between 20 to 60 years?

Streptococcus pneumoniae > Neisseria meningitidis > Haemophilus influenza

Adults older than 60 years?

Streptococcus pneumoniae > Listeria monocytogenes

What are the signs and symptoms of acute bacterial meningitis in adults?

Fever, nuchal rigidity, change in mental status (confusion and lethargy), headache (severe and generalized), seizures, focal neurologic deficits

What is the sensitivity of having at least one of the classic findings of fever, neck stiffness, and altered mental status for diagnosing bacterial meningitis?

99%

Does the absence of all three of these findings exclude the presence of bacterial meningitis?

Typically yes

What are Kernig and Brudzinski signs, which are sometimes seen in meningitis?

Kernig sign: with the patient supine and hip and knee flexed to 90°, the patient resists full extension of the knee

Brudzinski sign: spontaneous hip flexion while passively flexing the neck

What are the relative contraindications for performing a lumbar puncture in patients with suspected meningitis?

Mass effect on neuroimaging, thrombocytopenia, and spinal epidural abscess. All other patients with suspected meningitis should have cerebrospinal fluid obtained.

According to the Infectious Diseases Society of America, which patients should have a head CT scan before performing a lumbar puncture?

Immunocompromised state, history of central nervous system disease, new onset seizures, papilledema, abnormal level of consciousness, focal neurologic deficit

What are the typical lumbar puncture and cerebrospinal fluid (CSF) findings in acute bacterial meningitis?

Elevated opening pressure (>200 mm H_2O), white blood cell count is 1000-5000/mL with percentage of neutrophils >80%, elevated protein (100-500 mg/dL), low glucose (<40 mg/dL with a CSF: serum glucose ratio of <0.4)

What is the overall mortality rate of bacterial meningitis?

25%

CHAPTER 10

Insomnia and Sleep Disorders

What is the definition of insomnia?

Unsatisfactory sleep that impairs daytime functioning

What are three criteria for diagnosing insomnia?

1. Presents with difficulty initiating sleep or maintaining sleep, or with sleep that is nonrestorative for at least 1 month
2. Occurs despite adequate opportunity and circumstances for sleep
3. Impaired sleep causes deficits in daytime activity

What groups of people have higher rates of insomnia?

Adult women; persons who are unemployed, divorced, widowed, or of lower SES

What are symptoms of impaired daytime function?

Fatigue, headaches, GI symptoms, sleepiness, poor attention/concentration, increased errors/accidents, reduced motivation, mood disturbance, or social dysfunction

What are common causes of acute insomnia (<30 days)?

Situation stress, environmental stressors, or death of a loved one

What are the initial categories of treatment options for insomnia?

Behavioral therapies including relaxation and cognitive therapy, exercise, sleep hygiene instruction, stimulus control therapy, sleep restriction therapy, medications

What are reasons to avoid the use of over-the-counter antihistamines for insomnia?

Residual drowsiness, reduced sleep quality, anticholinergic side effects, minimal effectiveness

What are examples of good sleep hygiene actions?

Maintain regular sleep schedule, avoid caffeine after lunch, avoid alcohol near bedtime, avoid smoking, decrease light and stimuli in bedroom, exercise for 20 minutes daily more than 4 hours prior to bedtime, avoid daytime naps, avoid large meals before bed, maintain same sleep and wake time, avoid excessive time in bed

What are contraindications to medications used to treat insomnia?

Pregnancy, excess alcohol consumption, renal or hepatic disease, pulmonary disease or sleep apnea, adults over 75

What classes of medications target GABA receptors and can be used to promote sleep?

Long-acting benzodiazepines, nonbenzodiazepines, melatonin agonists

What is the advantage of nonbenzodiazepines (eszopiclone, zaleplon, zolpidem) over benzodiazepines for the treatment of chronic insomnia?

Fewer adverse effects, decreased risk of dependency

What are common side effects of medications used to treat insomnia?

Daytime sedation, drowsiness, lightheadedness, cognitive impairment, dependence, night wandering

Patients with insomnia due to a circadian rhythm disorder may benefit from what therapies?

Melatonin, phototherapy or chronotherapy

Before considering medication or treatment of insomnia, what should you do?

Treat any medical condition, psychiatric illness, substance abuse or sleep disorder that is causing insomnia

In this type of insomnia, the person has conditioned anxiety around falling asleep or staying asleep and often has genetic vulnerability, medical disorders, psychiatric conditions, or acute stress.

Primary psychophysiologic insomnia

What are the common sleep problems in the following age groups.

Infants and toddlers

Night waking, bedtime resistance

Preschool-aged children

Difficulties falling asleep, night awakenings

Middle childhood

Bedtime resistance, sleep-related anxiety

Adolescents

Insomnia

What behavioral interventions are advised for the treatment of behavioral insomnia in children?

Consistent bedtime routines, systematic ignoring, counseling, bedtime fading, positive reinforcement, parent education

What are common examples of circadian rhythm sleep disorders?

Jet lag and shift work

What common medical conditions are associated with insomnia?

Pulmonary disease, pain, rheumatologic disease, ischemic heart disease, GERD, BPH, menopause, hyperthyroidism, diabetes mellitus, neurologic disease, and heart failure

Early morning awakening is the hallmark symptom of what condition?

Depression

What psychiatric conditions are associated with insomnia?

Depression, substance abuse, anxiety, posttraumatic stress disorder

What medications commonly cause insomnia?

Caffeine, appetite suppressants, calcium channel blockers, some antidepressants, prednisone

Shift work sleep disorder has been associated with what medical and psychiatric problems?

Gastrointestinal and cardiovascular symptoms, depression, and substance abuse

What is the name for a sleep-wake cycle longer than 24 hours, accompanied by difficulty falling asleep?

Delayed sleep phase syndrome

An older adult complains of falling asleep and waking up before the desired clock time. What is the diagnosis?

Advanced sleep phase syndrome

What is the difference between a patient with advanced sleep phase syndrome and depression?

Depression has decreased latency (longer time) to REM sleep

An urge to move the legs accompanied by painful, itching or creeping sensations in the legs when a patient lies down to fall asleep is suggestive of what syndrome?	Restless legs syndrome (RLS)
What lab tests should you do to identify possible secondary causes?	Serum ferritin, pregnancy test, serum chemistry to rule out uremia and diabetes
What is the differential diagnosis of RLS?	Nocturnal leg cramps, akathisia, peripheral neuropathy, vascular disease
What class of medications are first line for the treatment of RLS?	Dopaminergic agents such as pramiprexole, ropinirole, and pergolide
This disorder is characterized by rhythmic limb movements, usually lower legs, during sleep causing fragmentation of sleep.	Periodic limb movement disorder (nocturnal myoclonus)
Pauses in respiration during sleep accompanied by brief arousals and nocturnal hypoxemia, along with daytime deficits should suggest what diagnosis?	Obstructive sleep apnea
This diagnosis is confirmed by what study?	Polysomnography (sleep study)
What are risk factors for this condition?	Condition causing narrowing of upper airway, obesity, male sex, smoking, nighttime nasal congestion, family history of OSA, menopause
This condition increases the risk of what other problems?	Motor vehicle collisions, hypertension, cardiovascular disease, impaired neurocognitive function
What is the definition of the following.	
Apnea	Absence of airflow at nose and mouth for 10 seconds or more
Hypopnea	Greater than 50% reduction in airflow at nose and mouth for at least 10 seconds
What is the treatment of choice for obstructive sleep apnea?	Nasal continuous positive airway pressure (CPAP)

CHAPTER 11

Dizziness and Syncope

DIZZINESS

What is dizziness?

A subjective sensation of movement of the head and/or body (vertigo, presyncope, disequilibrium)

What are the common causes of dizziness?

Peripheral vestibular dysfunction (40%), presyncope or disequilibrium (25%), psychiatric disorders such as depression, anxiety, or somatization (15%), central vestibular lesion (10%), unknown cause (10%)

VERTIGO

What causes vertigo?

A dysfunction of a part of the vestibular system, including the inner ear, vestibular nerve, nuclei within the medulla, and the connections to the vestibular sections of the cerebellum

What is peripheral vertigo?

Vertigo that results from dysfunction of the inner ear or the vestibular nerve

What is central vertigo?

Vertigo that results from dysfunction of the vestibular nuclei within the medulla or connections to the cerebellum

How do these signs and symptoms differ for central and peripheral vertigo?

Imbalance

Imbalance is severe with central vertigo and mild to moderate with peripheral vertigo.

Hearing loss

Hearing loss is rare with central vertigo and common with peripheral vertigo.

Nonauditory neurologic deficits

Nonauditory neurologic deficits are common with central vertigo and rare with peripheral vertigo.

What conditions can cause peripheral vertigo?

Benign paroxysmal positional vertigo, vestibular neuritis, Meniere disease, Ramsay-Hunt syndrome (herpes zoster oticus), perilymphatic fistula, vestibular schwannoma, aminoglycoside toxicity, otitis media

What causes vestibular neuritis?

Viral or postviral disorder of the vestibular portion of the eighth cranial nerve

What are the clinical manifestations of vestibular neuritis?

Acute onset of vertigo, nausea, vomiting, gait instability, nystagmus

What is labyrinthitis?

When unilateral hearing loss accompanies vestibular neuritis

Can steroids be used to treat vestibular neuritis?

Yes. Steroids have been shown to improve vestibular function at 12 months (compared to placebo) in patients with vestibular neuritis or labyrinthitis.

What triad of symptoms is associated with Meniere disease?

Vertigo, hearing loss (low frequency initially), tinnitus

What conditions can cause central vertigo?

Migraines, brainstem ischemia, cerebellar infarction or hemorrhage, multiple sclerosis

BENIGN PAROXYSMAL POSITIONAL VERTIGO

What movements tend to trigger vertigo in benign paroxysmal positional vertigo (BPPV)?

Looking up while standing or sitting, getting up from bed (symptoms are often in the morning), rolling over in bed

What causes BPPV?	Calcium debris (canalithiasis) within the semicircular canals of the inner ear (often the posterior canal) that causes movement of the endolymph
Patients with BPPV commonly report ear pain, hearing loss, and tinnitus. True or false?	False. Ear pain, hearing loss, and tinnitus are uncommon with BPPV.
What is the name of the maneuver that is used to help confirm the diagnosis of BPPV?	Dix-Hallpike maneuver
Describe the Dix-Hallpike maneuver.	Have seated patient extend neck and rotate head 45° to one side. Then, rapidly place the patient supine so that the head hangs over the edge of the table (head remains rotated). Observe for nystagmus for 30 seconds. Return the patient to the upright seated position and observe for nystagmus for 30 seconds. Repeat the maneuver with the head rotated 45° to the other side.
What indicates a positive test?	Nystagmus and vertigo
Does a negative test rule out BPPV?	No. The Dix-Hallpike maneuver does not reliably reproduce symptoms in all patients.
The nystagmus associated with BPPV is fatigable. True or false?	True. Multiple repetitions of the test will result in less nystagmus. Also, the nystagmus elicited by the Dix-Hallpike maneuver can be delayed.
What maneuvers can treat BPPV?	The Epley and Semont maneuvers
How long do BPPV symptoms persist without treatment?	Symptoms in patients with untreated posterior canal BPPV last for approximately a month before resolving spontaneously.

PRESYNCOPE/SYNCOPE

What is syncope?	A transient loss of consciousness that is associated with loss of postural tone with a spontaneous, immediate return to baseline neurologic function

What term is used to describe the symptom of "nearly blacking out" or "nearly fainting?"

Presyncope

The evaluation of presyncope is the same as the evaluation of syncope. True or false?

True

What are the common causes of syncope?

Vasovagal syncope (58%), cardiac conditions (23%), neurologic or psychiatric conditions (1%), unknown cause (18%)

What are life-threatening causes of syncope?

Cardiac conditions, bleeding, pulmonary embolism, subarachnoid hemorrhage

What cardiac conditions can cause syncope?

Arrhythmias (eg, bradycardia, AV nodal block, sustained ventricular tachycardia, supraventricular tachycardia), valvular disease, structural disease (eg, hypertrophic cardiomyopathy), tamponade, pacemaker malfunction

What is another name for neurocardiogenic syncope?

Vasovagal syncope

What is the pathophysiology of vasovagal syncope?

Increased vagal tone leads to bradycardia and/or vasodilation

Most patients with vasovagal syncope have a prodrome of lightheadedness, a sensation of warmth, pallor, diaphoresis, and nausea. True or false?

True. These symptoms result from increased vagal tone.

What are some common triggers for vasovagal syncope?

Micturition, defecation, deglutition, painful stimuli, fear or anxiety provoking situations (such as having blood drawn), prolonged standing, extreme emotions, heat exposure

What variant of vasovagal syncope results from pressure at the carotid sinus (eg, turning of the head, shaving, wearing a shirt with a tight collar)?

Carotid sinus hypersensitivity

What is the definition of orthostatic hypotension?

A symptomatic drop in blood pressure (BP) that occurs with changes in position

How do you test for orthostatic hypotension?

The posture test will demonstrate a systolic BP decrease of more than 20 mm Hg or a diastolic BP decrease of more than 10 mm Hg within 3 minutes of standing upright or sitting from a supine position. An increase in heart rate of 20 beats per minute is also commonly seen.

What conditions can cause orthostatic hypotension?

Hypovolemia, anemia, autonomic nervous system dysfunction (from Parkinson or diabetes mellitus), medications (such as antidepressants or antihypertensives)

Is stroke a common cause of syncope?

No. Stroke and transient ischemic attacks typically cause neurologic deficits that are not rapidly reversible.

CHAPTER 12

Red Eye and Eye Pain

What is the most common cause of red eye?	Conjunctivitis
What are other causes of red eye?	Keratitis, uveitis (iritis), scleritis, episcleritis, corneal abrasion, glaucoma, blepharitis, subconjunctival hemorrhage, foreign body
What key issues should be addressed in the patient's history when working up red eye?	Symptom duration, unilateral or bilateral involvement, quality and quantity of discharge, visual changes, severity of pain, photophobia, history of recent eye infection/allergies and treatment, personal or family history of autoimmune disease, contact-lens use

CONJUNCTIVITIS

What are the etiologies of conjunctivitis?	Infectious: bacterial, viral, chlamydial Noninfectious: allergies, irritants
A 15-year-old boy with asthma, eczema, and seasonal rhinitis presents with *itchy*, watery eyes. What is the most likely diagnosis?	Allergic conjunctivitis
What nonpharmacologic measures can help manage allergic conjunctivitis?	Allergen avoidance, avoidance of rubbing eyes which can cause mechanical mast cell degranulation, reduction of contact lens use (allergens can adhere to contact lens surfaces)
What kinds of eye drops help relieve allergic conjunctivitis?	Artificial tears (dilute allergens), antihistamine eye drops (olopatadine)

What is the disadvantage of oral antihistamines versus antihistamine eye drops?	The onset of action of oral antihistamines is longer than antihistamine eye drops; oral antihistamines cause systemic side effects, such as drowsiness.
Although not always reliable, what differences in examination findings might you expect in bacterial versus viral conjunctivitis?	Bacterial: opaque, thick, purulent discharge that reappears shortly after wiping the lids Viral: watery discharge

VIRAL CONJUNCTIVITIS

What are the offending microorganisms responsible for viral conjunctivitis?	Adenovirus (most common), enterovirus, coxsackievirus, varicella-zoster virus, Epstein-Barr virus, herpes simplex virus, influenza
What physical exam findings suggest viral conjunctivitis?	Minimal pain, diffuse conjunctival injection, mild itching, watery discharge, vision preserved, unaffected pupils, preauricular lymphadenopathy
What is the management of viral conjunctivitis?	Patient education about transmission, promote strict hand washing and discourage sharing of personal items, supportive treatment with cold compresses and artificial tears, topical antibiotics (rarely necessary because secondary bacterial infections are uncommon)
What is herpes zoster ophthalmicus?	Vesicular rash, keratitis, and uveitis caused by herpes zoster. Unilateral pain and tingling precede conjunctivitis and dermatomal rash. Early diagnosis can prevent corneal involvement and potential vision loss.
In herpes zoster, what cranial nerve would have to be affected to impair the patient's vision?	The frontal branch of the first division of the trigeminal nerve (V1)
What physical exam finding makes you suspect zoster involvement of the frontal branch of V1?	Vesicles involving the tip of the nose (Hutchinson sign)

What is the treatment of herpes zoster ophthalmicus?	Antiviral therapy, topical steroid drops to control keratitis and iritis, typically treated by ophthalmology

BACTERIAL CONJUNCTIVITIS

What are the three subtypes of bacterial conjunctivitis?	1. Acute (lasts up to 3-4 weeks) 2. Chronic (lasts more than 4 weeks) 3. Hyperacute (sudden onset and rapid progression)
What are the offending microorganisms responsible for acute and chronic bacterial conjunctivitis?	Children: *Streptococcus pneumoniae, Haemophilus influenzae* Adults: *Staphylococcus aureus, Moraxella* species, *Escherichia coli, Pseudomonas* species
What is the offending pathogen responsible for hyperacute bacterial conjunctivitis?	*Neisseria gonorrhoeae*
What is the best clinical predictor when considering a diagnosis of bacterial conjunctivitis?	Profuse, thick mucopurulent secretions
What is the treatment of acute bacterial conjunctivitis?	Antibiotic eye drops or ointment 4-6 times a day though studies have indicated that most cases are self-limited; frequent hand washing to prevent spreading; for cases lasting greater than 4 weeks, refer to ophthalmology for management of chronic bacterial conjunctivitis
Sudden onset of profuse, purulent discharge accompanied by intense hyperemia of conjunctiva in a sexually active patient suggests what process?	Hyperacute gonococcal conjunctivitis
What is the treatment of hyperacute bacterial conjunctivitis?	Danger of rapid progression and potential corneal perforation requires aggressive management by an ophthalmologist and possible hospitalization, systemic antibiotics +/− topical therapy, frequent eye irrigation

A patient returns to your office with no response to standard antibacterial treatment for a suspected acute bacterial conjunctivitis. Given that the patient is sexually active, what other diagnoses and treatment might you pursue at this stage?

Chlamydial conjunctivitis (signs and symptoms which do not resolve with standard antibiotic therapy); treat topically with erythromycin ophthalmic ointment; treat possible genital infection with azithromycin or doxycycline; encourage treatment for patient's sexual partner(s)

What are the three types of neonatal conjunctivitis?

1. Chemical (less than 24 hours old)
2. Gonorrheal (2-5 days old)
3. Chlamydial (5-14 days old)

Erythromycin ointment is given prophylactically to all newborns at birth to decrease the risk of what type of neonatal conjunctivitis?

Gonococcal conjunctivitis

Twelve hours after a newborn receives her erythromycin drops she develops redness in both eyes and a nonpurulent discharge. What is the most likely diagnosis?

Chemical conjunctivitis precipitated by the erythromycin drops; will resolve in 48 hours

What is the typical presentation of neonatal gonococcal conjunctivitis?

Profuse, purulent discharge and striking hyperemia and edema 2-5 days after birth

What is the treatment?

Topical and systemic antibiotics (penicillin, ceftriaxone, or azithromycin)

What is the most common cause of neonatal conjunctivitis?

Chlamydia (transmission during passage in birth canal)

What is the treatment for neonatal chlamydial conjunctivitis?

Topical tetracycline and oral erythromycin

What is the role of the systemic antibiotic component of neonatal conjunctival therapy?

To prevent chlamydial pneumonia

What should you suspect in a school-aged child who presents with features of gonococcal conjunctivitis?

Sexual abuse

UVEITIS AND KERATITIS

What is the most likely diagnosis in a patient with ocular pain, photophobia, ciliary flush (ring of redness around the iris), and lack of foreign body sensation?

Uveitis (the uvea includes the iris, ciliary body, and choroids)

What systemic inflammatory illnesses are associated with uveitis?

Ankylosing spondylitis, Reiter syndrome, psoriatic arthritis, inflammatory bowel disease (IBD), sarcoidosis, Behcet disease, juvenile rheumatoid arthritis, multiple sclerosis, Kawasaki disease, systemic lupus erythematosus (SLE), systemic vasculitis

What are the most common pathogens which cause uveitis in a non-compromised host?

Toxoplasma gondii, Bartonella henselae (cat scratch disease), *Treponema pallidum* (syphilis), West Nile virus

What are the most common infectious causes of uveitis in an immunocompromised host?

Cytomegalovirus (CMV), tuberculosis

What complications can be seen with untreated uveitis?

Glaucoma and cataracts; refer to ophthalmology if uveitis is suspected

What is keratitis?

Inflammation of the cornea

How does the presentation of keratitis overlap with and differ from uveitis?

Like uveitis, keratitis can cause red eye and photophobia. Unlike uveitis, keratitis can cause foreign body sensation, a corneal opacity on exam, and exhibit fluorescein uptake.

Wearing contacts overnight can increase the risk of developing keratitis. True or false?

True

CORNEAL ABRASION

What are the common mechanisms of corneal injury?

Trauma, infection, contact lenses worn for long periods, excessive exposure to ultraviolet light

What signs and symptoms are seen with corneal abrasions?

Eye pain, inability to open eyelid secondary to foreign body sensation

In cases of suspected corneal abrasion, what is the best method of examination?

Fluorescein dye and Wood lamp

Eye patching hastens the resolution of corneal abrasions. True or false?

False. Patching was thought to promote healing by keeping the eyelid stationary over the defect; however, studies have not demonstrated that the practice improves outcomes.

What is the treatment of corneal abrasions?

Antibiotic eye drops to prevent superinfection though the practice has not been well studied

GLAUCOMA

What disease process is described as a progressive "tunneling" visual field loss usually associated with an increase in intraocular pressure that compresses the optic nerve over time?

Open-angle glaucoma

What are the risk factors for open-angle glaucoma?

Elevated intraocular pressure, family history, advanced age, African American ethnicity, myopia

What glaucoma medications used to treat open-angle glaucoma decrease the production of aqueous humor?

Alpha-adrenergic agonists, beta-adrenergic blockers, carbonic anhydrase inhibitors, cholinergic agonists

What glaucoma medications used to treat open-angle glaucoma increase the outflow of aqueous humor?

Alpha-adrenergic agonists, miotics, epinephrine compounds, prostaglandins

An elderly lady complains of an abruptly painful, red eye with decreased vision and halos around lights as well as nausea and vomiting. Examination shows intense redness around the cornea with corneal haze and a fixed, unreactive pupil. What is the diagnosis?

Acute angle-closure glaucoma

| How do you treat acute angle-closure glaucoma until the ophthalmologist is reached? | An antiemetic, two 250-mg oral tablets of acetazolamide, and topical agents (alpha-adrenergic agonists, beta-adrenergic blockers, carbonic anhydrase inhibitors, cholinergic agonists) to decrease intraocular pressure |

EYELID DISORDERS

What are common eyelid disorders which may present with redness?	Blepharitis, styes, chalazions
What is a stye?	A tender, erythematous nodule that arises acutely from inflammation of meibomian glands at the lid margin
What do patients typically complain of with a stye?	Waking up in the morning with a red, painful bump at the lid margin
What is the treatment of styes?	Apply warm compresses for 15 minutes four times daily; antibiotic ointments are frequently used though studies to support this practice are lacking.
Will styes go away on their own?	Yes. They typically resolve spontaneously.
What is a chalazion?	A painless nodule around the lid margin arising from chronic inflammation of a meibomian gland; styes can occasionally harden into chalazions
What is the initial treatment of chalazions?	Warm compresses (since this is a granulomatous condition, antibiotics do not help)
Will chalazions go away on their own?	Usually, but they may require incision and curettage under local anesthesia if they do not resolve after 3-4 weeks
What is blepharitis?	Inflammation of the eyelid characterized by scaling and redness along the lid margins
What are the underlying causes of blepharitis?	Staphylococcal infection, scalp seborrhea, acne rosacea

What is the treatment for blepharitis?   Warm compresses, eyelid margin scrubs, topical antibiotics, antidandruff shampoos

What are xanthomas?   These are painless, yellowish nodules often occurring on the eyelids and can be associated with dyslipidemia.

ORBITAL CELLULITIS

What is orbital cellulitis?   A sight-threatening infection of the fat and muscle contained within the bony orbit

What are the symptoms associated with orbital cellulitis?   Pain with movement of the eye, redness, swelling, blurry vision, double vision

What are the signs of orbital cellulitis?   Edema (especially conjunctival), erythema, limitations of eye movement, vision loss

What is the most common risk factor for orbital cellulitis?   History of sinusitis

What age group is most commonly affected by orbital cellulitis?   Children

What are the most common causative microorganisms?   Streptococci, *S. aureus*, non-spore forming anaerobes, mixed infection (often hard to identify)

What is the appropriate workup of a patient with suspected orbital cellulitis?   Prompt imaging of the orbit to determine the extent of inflammation and the presence of orbital or subperiosteal abscesses

What are the signs of an orbital abscess?   Unilateral ophthalmoplegia, impairment of vision, conjunctival swelling

What is the treatment of orbital cellulitis?   Start IV broad-spectrum antibiotics; consider referral for possible orbital surgery

Why is the incidence of orbital cellulitis decreasing?   *H. influenzae* type B (HIB) vaccine

CHAPTER 13

Ear, Nose, and Throat Complaints

NASAL CONGESTION

What is the most common cause of chronic rhinitis and nasal congestion?	Allergic rhinitis
What is the most common cause of acute rhinitis and nasal congestion (and also happens to be the leading cause of work and school absenteeism)?	The common cold
What are some other causes of rhinitis and nasal congestion?	Other upper respiratory infections (influenza, rhinosinusitis), allergic rhinitis, idiopathic rhinitis (ie, vasomotor rhinitis, autonomic hyperresponsiveness), atrophic rhinitis, rhinitis medicamentosum from drug withdrawal (eg, cocaine, OTC decongestant nasal sprays), nasal foreign bodies
What is rhinosinusitis (aka "sinusitis")?	Inflammation of one or more of the paranasal sinuses
How does it develop?	Nasal passage edema (usually due to infection) causes obstruction of the sinus ostia
What symptoms distinguish the following ailments: common cold, influenza, sinusitis, allergic rhinitis?	Refer to the table on next page:

Symptoms of Common Upper Respiratory Ailments

	Fever	Headache or Facial Pain	Orbital Symptoms	Myalgias	Weakness and Fatigue	Nasal Symptoms	Throat Symptoms/ Cough/Other Symptoms[a]
Common cold	Mild, if present	Not usually present	None	Not usual	Not usual	Nasal congestion, sneezing	Postnasal drip with sore throat and cough
Influenza	High fever	Headache is prominent	None	Moderate to severe	Moderate to severe	Sometimes nasal congestion and sneezing are present	Sore throat is sometimes present; cough is common and often severe with significant chest discomfort; may have diarrhea and vomiting

Sinusitis	Sometimes present	Often present with pressure or pain over sinuses; headache often worse when leaning forward	Pressure around eyes and periorbital edema (beware of orbital complications) especially when ethmoid sinus involved	Not usual	Fatigue sometimes present	Thick, yellow, sometimes foul-smelling discharge; nasal obstruction; decreased or absent ability to smell	Postnasal drip may cause sore throat and cough, especially at night; halitosis; painful mastication
Allergic rhinitis	Never	Present if allergies are causing significant sinus congestion	Itchy, watery eyes often present	Never	Never	Exposure to allergen often causes profuse and watery rhinorrhea	Postnasal drip may cause throat discomfort ("itchiness"), cough, asthma exacerbation

aRefer to questions about disease-specific complications for details regarding symptoms present in severe disease

What kind of pathogen is the most common cause of the common cold and how is it most commonly transmitted?

Viruses (eg, rhinovirus, coronavirus) transmitted by hand-to-hand contact

How long do colds last?

A few days to a few weeks (this is important to tell patients)

What are the potential complications of a cold?

Sinusitis, otitis media, lower respiratory tract infection, exacerbation of asthma/ chronic obstructive pulmonary disease (COPD)

What are some nonpharmacologic ways to help relieve cold symptoms?

Rest, high fluid intake, saline drops, humidifier

What over-the-counter medications can be used for symptomatic relief of cold symptoms?

Acetaminophen or ibuprofen for fever and headache, pseudoephedrine for congestion and rhinorrhea, dextromethorphan/guaifenesin for cough

Of the three genera of influenza viruses (A, B, and C) which is the most virulent and has been the cause of all pandemics, including the 1918 Spanish Flu Pandemic and the 2009 H1N1 Flu Pandemic?

Influenza A

What are the main prevention strategies for the flu?

Good hygiene (especially effective hand washing), flu vaccine (intramuscular or nasal)

What are the pharmacologic treatments for the flu and within what timeframe from the onset of symptoms should they be administered?

Oseltamivir (oral) and zanamivir (inhaled), both of which are neuraminidase inhibitors. Treatment should be initiated within 48 hours of the onset of symptoms. Treatments can be used in patients who have been ill greater than 48 hours if they have severe disease requiring hospitalization.

What are the major complications of the flu?

Pneumonia (primary influenza pneumonia, *S. aureus* pneumonia), sometimes requiring supplemental oxygen or mechanical ventilation, cardiopulmonary insufficiency (shock, organ failure), myocarditis, rhabdomyolysis, neurologic impairment or disease (altered mental status, encephalitis), exacerbation of chronic conditions

Name the four sinus cavities.	1. Ethmoid 2. Maxillary 3. Frontal 4. Sphenoid
Which of these are present at birth?	Ethmoid and maxillary
Which begins development at age 2 years but is only apparent by x-ray at 5 years?	Sphenoid
Which is the last to develop?	Frontal (develops from age 4-20 years)
Why is the order of sinus development important?	In children, most infections involve the ethmoid and maxillary sinuses; frontal and sphenoid infections usually begin to appear in adolescence
Children with sinusitis often complain of headache and facial pain. True or false?	False. Remember the location of the earlier developing sinuses.
During what season does the incidence of sinusitis peak?	Winter
Under what circumstance does fungal sinusitis develop?	Immunocompromised patient. Look for mucormycosis (*Mucor, Rhizopus*) in diabetics.
What findings may help distinguish a bacterial sinusitis from a viral one?	Bacterial sinusitis is more likely to present with at least one of the following: fever, unilateral sinus pain, maxillary tooth pain, persistence of symptoms for greater than 7-10 days, "double sickening" (aka biphasic illness).
What is the "double sickening" phenomenon?	Biphasic illness: patient begins to improve from a URI (upper respiratory infection) but then acquires a secondary bacterial acute sinusitis
What is the duration of acute versus subacute versus chronic sinusitis?	Acute: greater than 3 days but less than 4 weeks Subacute: 4-12 weeks Chronic: greater than 12 weeks
What are the usual bacterial causes of acute sinusitis versus chronic sinusitis?	Acute: *Streptococcus pneumoniae, Haemophilus influenzae, Moraxella catarrhalis,* or *Staphylococcus aureus* Chronic: anaerobic bacteria

What kinds of pathogens are the usual causes of sinusitis when it results from a spreading dental infection?

Microaerophilic or anaerobic bacteria

Most cases of sinusitis will spontaneously resolve without antibiotics within 2 weeks. True or false?

True

Under what circumstances should you consider the use of antibiotics to treat sinusitis?

Antibiotic use recommendations for sinusitis are ever-changing. However, in general, patients who have sinusitis that is likely bacterial and those without symptom improvement for more than 7-14 days *may* benefit from antibiotics (sometimes risk of drug side effects is greater than benefits).

Under what circumstances should you consider intravenous (IV) antibiotics to treat sinusitis?

Patients with very severe symptoms or signs of complications (eg, facial erythema, orbital manifestations)

What is the initial treatment of acute sinusitis?

Nonpharmacologic treatment: saline nasal sprays, humidifier

Nasal symptom relief: decongestants, nasal steroids, and antihistamines (efficacy is controversial)

Pain relief: analgesics (eg, acetaminophen, ibuprofen)

What antibiotics are used to treat bacterial sinusitis?

High-dose amoxicillin, amoxicillin-clavulanate, cephalosporins, macrolides. Because of changes in drug-resistance, check your most updated antibiotic handbook for guidance.

What systemic diseases may predispose a patient to recurrent or persistent sinusitis?

Cystic fibrosis, Kartagener syndrome, rare vasculitides (eg, Wegener granulomatosus, Churg-Strauss syndrome), immune deficiency (including diabetes)

What circumstances dictate an otolaryngology consultation (for possible surgery) for the treatment of sinusitis?

Patients with more than three attacks in 1 year, chronic sinusitis, unresponsiveness to antibiotics, anatomic abnormalities amenable to surgery

Are imaging studies helpful in the initial evaluation of sinusitis?

No (except in uncertain or recurrent cases)

Under what circumstances is a CT scan indicated?	To establish a diagnosis of chronic sinusitis, work up a preoperative patient, or obtain more information when medical management has failed.
What are the potential complications of sinusitis?	Mucocele or mucopyoceles, preseptal or orbital cellulitis, orbital or brain abscess, cavernous or sagittal sinus thrombosis, meningitis, encephalitis, subdural empyema, osteomyelitis. Note: a patient who exhibits ocular and or neural signs or symptoms should be evaluated and treated *promptly*.
In what sinus do mucoceles most frequently occur?	Frontal sinus
How does the patient present?	Displaced eye, diplopia
Orbital complications from sinusitis are most likely to happen when the infection is in what sinus cavity?	Ethmoid sinus
What are the signs of cavernous sinus thrombosis?	Bilateral ophthalmoplegia, conjunctival swelling, retinal engorgement, fever
What allergens typically cause seasonal allergies?	Pollens (from trees, grasses, weeds) and mold spores
What allergens typically cause perennial allergies?	Dust mites, mold spores, cockroach feces, pet dander
What is the primary "treatment" of allergic rhinitis?	Avoidance of allergens
Oral antihistamines usually help reduce what symptoms associated with allergic rhinitis?	Sneezing, rhinorrhea
Are antihistamines effective in relieving nasal congestion?	No. Generally, decongestants are needed *in addition* to antihistamines in order to relieve congestion.
What are some available second-generation antihistamines?	Loratadine, desloratadine, fexofenadine, cetirizine

What are the main differences between first- and second-generation antihistamines?

Second-generation antihistamines are less likely to cause anticholinergic side effects (eg, drowsiness), and some come in an antihistamine-decongestant combination; they are not necessarily more effective, but are more expensive and sometimes require a prescription.

What types of nasal sprays are available for the treatment of allergic rhinitis?

Steroid nasal sprays (beclomethasone, flunisolide, fluticasone propionate, fluticasone furoate, mometasone, triamcinolone, budesonide), anti-histamine spray (azelastine), mast cell stabilizer (cromolyn sodium), anticholinergic agents (eg, ipratropium bromide)

Which type of nasal spray relieves rhinorrhea but does not relieve nasal congestion or sneezing?

Anticholinergic spray

Which of the steroid nasal sprays is effective in relieving allergic eye symptoms in addition to nasal symptoms?

Fluticasone furoate

All nasal sprays are more effective when used consistently, not simply in response to symptoms when they arise; however, which type of nasal spray *never works* once allergy symptoms are already present and must always be used prior to allergen exposure?

Mast cell stabilizer

Which nasal sprays are approved for children less than 6 years old?

Azelastine (5 years), mometasone (2 years), fluticasone furoate (2 years), fluticasone propionate (4 years)

What techniques should patients employ when administering nasal sprays?

First blow nose to remove mucus from nasal passages, shake bottle before removing the cap, sniff gently while spraying with tip of bottle pointing to outer part of nostril.

Which patients should undergo allergen skin testing?

Patients with moderate to severe symptoms or perennial allergies, patients who have failed medical treatment, patients who need guidance for appropriate avoidance measures or immunotherapy

What medications should be withheld before allergen skin testing?	Methylxanthines, beta-blockers, antihistamines
What does radioallergosorbent (RAST) testing measure?	Allergen-specific IgE levels
What is immunotherapy (also known as desensitization)?	Patient receives weekly injections with gradually increasing doses of antigens and over time the IgE response diminishes.
What class of antihypertensives should be avoided during immunotherapy?	Beta-blockers
How long should immunotherapy be administered to avoid recurrence of symptoms?	3-5 years

NOSEBLEEDS

What is the most common cause of nosebleeds (epistaxis)?	Local trauma caused by nose picking or direct blunt trauma
What are some other causes of epistaxis?	• Other trauma (surgery, forceful blowing) • Chronic irritation (dry air, smoke/pollutants) • Cocaine use • Intranasal medications • Nasal foreign body • Intranasal polyp or tumor • Systemic problems: bleeding diathesis, blood thinning medications, hypertension
What accompanying symptoms would prompt an evaluation for bleeding disorders?	Frequent bleeding or bleeding from multiple sites other than just the nose (excessive bleeding/bruising from minor wounds, bleeding gums, hematemesis, melena, menorrhagia, history of post-partum bleeding, history of excessive bleeding during surgery, etc)
What labs would you obtain to start this evaluation?	Complete blood count, prothrombin time (PT) and international normalized ratio (INR), partial thromboplastin time (PTT), peripheral blood smear

What is Kiesselbach plexus?

An area in the anteroinferior part of the nasal septum where several arteries anastomose and is the most frequent area of epistaxis

What is the management of a stable patient with a nosebleed?

Patient should lean forward (avoids posterior blood accumulation), blow out clots, then squeeze cartilaginous nose (steady moderate pressure for 5-20 minutes) while you perform history and physical (look for easily reversible cause of bleeding).

If the above does not work and you confirm an anterior nosebleed with direct visualization, what other steps can you take to stop the bleeding?

Intranasal oxymetazoline (decongestant) and lidocaine (analgesic) plus phenylephrine, cautery with silver nitrate, or nasal packing

If a patient is bleeding profusely and the bleeding is difficult to stop, what kind of bleed (in terms of location) are you most likely dealing with?

Posterior bleed (although anterior bleed is still possible)

What additional management steps should you take for a bleed of this magnitude?

- Use universal precautions (eye mask, gown)
- Start large bore IV
- Stat orders: CBC, type and cross, epistaxis tray
- Tamponade bleed: nasal catheter with dual-chambered cuff (least complicated method), Foley catheter, or posterior nasal packing
- Consider otolaryngology consult

What are the most worrisome complications from severe acute nosebleeds?

Airway compromise and hemodynamic instability

EARACHE

What is acute otitis media (AOM)?

Middle ear inflammation associated with an infection

How is AOM thought to develop?

Dysfunction and/or inflammation of the eustachian tube causes inadequate ventilation of the middle ear resulting in a negative pressure that pulls up fluid and infectious agents.

Name the causes of eustachian tube dysfunction/inflammation.

URI, allergies, enlarged adenoids, irritants (ie, tobacco smoke), genetic factors

What are the symptoms?

Earache, decreased hearing, fever, nausea, vomiting

Why are symptoms alone not enough to make a diagnosis?

There is no one symptom that is found reliably in all patients with AOM.

What does visualization of the tympanic membrane (TM) reveal?

Bulging, red, dull, or opaque TM; displaced or absent light reflex; loss of bony landmarks; impaired TM mobility

Which of these is the most important in diagnosis?

TM mobility

Does an erythematous TM indicate AOM?

Not necessarily. Increased intravascular pressure can also cause the TM to redden, such as when a child is crying.

What is the peak age of onset of AOM?

6 months to 7 years

What is the peak season of AOM?

Winter, because of increased upper respiratory infections

What are the most common bacterial causes of AOM?

S. pneumoniae, H. influenzae, M. catarrhalis

What is the treatment for AOM?

Analgesic and antibiotic

What is the first-line antibiotic?

High-dose amoxicillin (for children, this means 70-90 mg/kg/day vs. standard 40 mg/kg/day)

Children under what age should be treated with antibiotics if AOM is suspected?

Children under 6 months should always be treated. Children between 6 and 24 months should be treated with antibiotics unless the child has very mild disease.

What is the rationale for the "watch and wait" approach of AOM in children over 24 months?

While severe disease should always be treated with antibiotics immediately regardless of age, most AOM is not severe and will resolve spontaneously. Treatment only needs to consist of pain management.

Almost every AOM is followed by otitis media with effusion (fluid in the middle ear). How long may it take for the effusion to clear?

Up to 3 months

By definition, what is recurrent otitis media?	Three or more episodes of acute AOM in a 6-month period or four or more in 12 months
What are the treatment options?	Antibiotic prophylaxis or surgery (tympanostomy tubes)
What antibiotics can be used for prophylaxis?	Amoxicillin and sulfisoxazole
How do tympanostomy tubes help manage AOM recurrence?	They decrease recurrence by ventilating and equalizing pressure in the middle ear. When recurrence does occur, they enable the use of topical antibiotics.
What are the complications of AOM?	Hearing loss, mastoiditis, cholesteatoma, CNS infections, thrombosis
What is otitis externa (OE)?	Inflammation of the ear canal, usually caused by infection ("swimmer's ear")
What is the peak season of OE?	Summer
What are the risk factors for developing OE?	Excessive exposure to water (strips cerumen, elevates pH), excessive manipulation of ear canal (cotton swabs), chronic dermatologic condition, immune dysfunction
What are the signs and symptoms of OE?	Earache, canal is red and edematous and has purulent drainage, movement of tragus is very painful
What are the most common bacterial causes of OE?	Pseudomonas sp., *S. aureus*, *Staphylococcus epidermidis*
What ear drops may be used to treat bacterial OE?	2% acetic acid solution or antibiotic (neomycin, polymyxin B, ciprofloxacin, ofloxacin, gentamicin, tobramycin) drops with or without hydrocortisone
Which antibiotic is FDA-approved for use when the tympanic membrane is ruptured?	Ofloxacin
What is the treatment of fungal OE?	Topical clotrimazole, tolnaftate, or oral fluconazole
What nonpharmacologic strategies help the patient prevent OE recurrences?	Drying canals with alcohol drops (1/3 white vinegar, 2/3 rubbing alcohol), then acidifying with 2% acetic acid solution

What is malignant otitis externa?	Invasive cellulitis around the ear most often occurring in diabetics and immune compromised patients (HIV, chemotherapy)
What causes it?	*Pseudomonas aeruginosa* in greater than 90%
How is it treated?	Ciprofloxacin (early disease), IV antibiotics, surgical debridement (severe disease)
Why should you scan the patient's head (either CT or MRI)?	To rule out osteomyelitis

TINNITUS

What is tinnitus?	The perception of sound when there is no actual *external* acoustic signal. The patient may describe any number of sounds including humming, clicking, whistling, pulsatile whoozing, etc.
What is the difference between objective tinnitus and subjective tinnitus?	Objective tinnitus means the sound the patient hears is an actual sound coming from within the head/neck (such as a bruit); in subjective tinnitus no actual sound is occurring (more common than objective tinnitus).
What are some common causes of tinnitus?	Noise-induced hearing loss, Meniere disease, acoustic neuroma, ototoxic medications (chemotherapy, aminoglycosides, some diuretics, etc), multiple sclerosis, depression and anxiety
What is the most common cause of tinnitus?	Noise-induced hearing loss
What are the basic first steps in the evaluation of tinnitus?	Perform history and physical focused on diseases of the ear and causes of objective tinnitus (such as a bruit); order an audiogram to assess for hearing loss
What is the most worrisome cause of *unilateral* tinnitus?	Acoustic neuroma

What is the most common cause of medication-induced tinnitus and what is the treatment? — Aspirin and aspirin-containing products. Discontinuation of product resolves tinnitus.

For most patients with mild to moderate tinnitus, what simple conservative measures achieve some symptom improvement (or at least prevent worsening)? — Avoid hazardous noise (if exposure is necessary, wear proper ear protection), limit caffeine intake, avoid silence (keep a low level of background noise, such as a fan), manage stress.

What imaging would you order if you suspect that a patient has a pulsatile tinnitus of vascular origin? — MRI/MRA

SORE THROAT

What is pharyngitis? — Inflammation of the pharynx, hypopharynx, uvula, or tonsils

What are some noninfectious causes of pharyngitis? — Trauma, smoke inhalation, pollutants, allergies, gastroesophageal reflux

What is the most common infectious cause of pharyngitis? — Adenovirus

What other viruses can cause pharyngitis? — Rhinovirus, coxsackievirus, herpesvirus (Epstein-Barr virus, herpes simplex virus, varicella virus)

Describe hand, foot, and mouth disease (caused by a coxsackievirus). — Erythematous-based small vesicles or ulcers in the pharynx and on the palms and soles

Describe the oral lesions caused by herpes simplex virus. — Shallow, erythematous-based small vesicles; ulcers on the gingival, vermillion border, and/or pharynx

Exudative tonsillitis, pharyngitis (for more than 10-14 days), cervical lymphadenopathy, fever, fatigue, and hepatosplenomegaly are characteristic of what common cause of pharyngitis? — Infectious mononucleosis. It is caused by Epstein-Barr virus but other viruses (cytomegalovirus) may cause a mononucleosis-like syndrome.

What test can be used to diagnose infectious mononucleosis? — Monospot test (detects heterophile antibodies)

What other tests should be performed in patients with infectious mononucleosis?

Liver function tests, complete blood count (CBC) and platelets, Coombs test

What are the complications of infectious mononucleosis?

Hepatitis, ruptured spleen, low blood cell counts, CNS infections

What precaution should patients take to reduce the risk of splenic rupture?

Avoid contact sports and heavy lifting in the first 2-3 weeks of illness

Which antibiotics can cause a rash in patients with infectious mononucleosis?

Amoxicillin or ampicillin which are often given when a clinician mistakes mononucleosis for a streptococcal throat infection

In patients presenting with mononucleosis-like illness, why is it so important to take a social history?

Sexually transmitted infections (gonorrhea, chlamydia, HIV) may present with pharyngitis. Recognizing the similarities between primary HIV (acute retroviral syndrome) and infectious mononucleosis is particularly important since it increases the rate of early HIV detection.

Primary HIV typically presents within how many weeks of initial infection?

2-3 weeks

In primary HIV, how high is the viral load?

HIV viral load is greater than 10,000 copies/mL

Give some examples of nonviral pathogens that can cause pharyngitis?

Group A beta-hemolytic streptococcus (GABHS), *Chlamydophila pneumoniae*, *Mycoplasma*, *Corynebacterium diphtheriae*, *Neisseria gonorrhoeae*, *Candida*

In what season is GABHS most common?

Winter and early spring

A sore throat from GABHS infection lasts how long?

Less than a week (longer than that probably means that it is something else)

The Centor criteria are often used to distinguish GABHS from other causes of pharyngitis. What are the Centor criteria?

1. Tonsillar exudates
2. Tender anterior cervical adenopathy
3. Fever
4. Absence of cough

Note: use the one-point age modifier if it makes a difference in the score interpretation, add one point to the score for children <15 years, subtract one for adults >45 years.

What is the test of choice for diagnosing strep throat?

Rapid streptococcal antigen test

How does the Centor score help determine when a rapid strep test should be ordered and when antibiotics should be given?

A rapid strep test should be done when the Centor score is 2 or 3 and antibiotics should be used if the test is positive. A score of 4 or 5 should be treated with empiric antibiotics. A score of 0 or 1 does not need rapid strep testing or antibiotics.

What test should be done if the rapid strep test is negative but clinical suspicion remains high?

Throat culture on blood agar plate (BAP)

What is the preferred treatment for GABHS and why?

Oral penicillin V potassium for 10 days or a one-time dose of intramuscular penicillin G benzathine. Penicillin is a low-cost, narrow-spectrum antibiotic, with long-proven efficacy.

What is the treatment if the patient has a penicillin allergy?

Macrolides (eg, azithromycin) or clindamycin

What is the rationale for treating GABHS?

Treatment can shorten illness duration (although usually only by one day), prevent rheumatic fever, and prevent peritonsillar abscess.

What are the complications of GABHS?

Rheumatic fever (and subsequent heart valve damage), peritonsillar abscess, acute poststreptococcal glomerulonephritis (APSGN)

What are some signs and symptoms of rheumatic fever?

Carditis, erythema marginatum, migratory polyarthritis, subcutaneous skin nodules, chorea, fever

What are the signs and symptoms of peritonsillar abscess?

Worsening sore throat, fever, odynophagia/dysphagia, difficulty speaking, large tonsils, displaced palate, deviated uvula, difficulty in neck extension, limited jaw movement

How is it treated?

Drainage (with 18-gauge needle or surgically) and antibiotics (clindamycin or second- or third-generation cephalosporin)

What are the signs and symptoms of APSGN?

Edema, hypertension, gross hematuria, oliguria. At least half of the patients are asymptomatic.

Can antibiotic treatment for GABHS prevent APSGN?

Evidence has not shown that antibiotic treatment can reduce the incidence of APSGN.

What is the typical latent period between GABHS infection and APSGN?

7-21 days (average = 10)

HOARSENESS

What is hoarseness?

A change in voice quality

What mucosal lesions can cause hoarseness in kids?

Vocal fold nodules and granulomas

What are causes of chronic laryngitis (lasting more than 3 months)?

Exposure to environmental irritants, allergies, chronic sinusitis, medications (such as inhaled steroids), gastroesophageal reflux, tumors (benign and malignant)

What is the most common laryngeal cancer in adults?

Squamous cell carcinoma (risk factors include tobacco and alcohol use)

What are causes of unilateral vocal fold paralysis from recurrent laryngeal nerve injury in adults?

Iatrogenic injury, extra-laryngeal malignancy (eg, thyroid cancer), degenerative neural disorders (eg, amyotrophic lateral sclerosis), demyelinating disease (eg, multiple sclerosis)

Bacterial infections are a more common cause of laryngitis than viral infections. True or false?

False. Laryngitis is typically from viral infections but secondary bacterial infections can occur (look for fever, purulent exudates, and progressive pain).

When hoarseness lasts for more than 2 weeks and does not have an apparent benign cause, a patient should undergo what kind of procedure?

Direct or indirect laryngoscopy

CHAPTER 14

Neck Mass

What is the greatest concern when an adult presents with a neck mass?	Malignancy (risk of malignancy increases with age)
What factors increase the likelihood of neck malignancy?	Smoking, heavy alcohol use, history of radiation treatment, chronic sun exposure, family history
What is the most common site of neck masses?	Lymph nodes
What are the most common congenital neck masses of the lateral neck?	Brachial anomalies (cyst, sinus, fistula)
What is the most common type of branchial anomaly and how does it typically present?	Second arch branchial cyst presenting in infants as a painless fluctuant mass in the anterior triangle
What is the most common congenital neck mass of the midline neck?	Thyroglossal duct cyst
What kind of malignancy has been reported within thyroglossal duct cysts?	Thyroid carcinoma
What signs and symptoms indicate that a neck mass is most likely due to an inflammatory process?	Recent infection, fever, tenderness and erythema at site of mass, rapidly growing
Viruses, bacteria, typical and atypical mycobacteria, parasites, and fungi can all cause infection leading to inflammatory neck masses. Which is the most common?	Viruses
What is the treatment for neck abscesses?	Surgical incision and drainage and/or intravenous (IV) antibiotics

What types of bacteria are the most common cause of neck masses?	*Staphylococcus* and *streptococcus* bacteria
What is the treatment?	10-day course of beta-lactamase resistant antibiotic
What pathogen causes cat scratch disease?	*Bartonella henselae*
What are the common clinical findings in cat scratch disease?	Large lymphadenopathy (usually unilateral) that enlarges or does not resolve, low grade fever, joint or muscle aches

To diagnose Kawasaki syndrome (vasculitis in children 5 years old or less) five of six criteria must be met, one of which is high fever for more than 5 days. What are the other five criteria?

1. Cervical adenopathy (at least 1.5 cm in diameter)
2. Conjunctival injection
3. Rednessof the oral cavity
4. Polymorphous exanthem
5. Reddening and/or swelling of the palms/soles (sometimes desquamation occurs)

What cardiovascular complication may arise from Kawasaki?	Coronary artery aneurysm
What is the treatment used to prevent the complications of Kawasaki?	IV immunoglobulin and aspirin (one of the few indications for aspirin use in children)
If a patient has a neck mass that by history is suggestive of an infectious process but has not responded to broad-spectrum antibiotic treatment, what tests should you order next?	PPD and chest x-ray
What is scrofula?	Neck lymphadenitis due to mycobacteria (including but not limited to tuberculosis)
How does it typically present?	As a single large cervical lymph node with an overlying violaceous color appearing later; strongly reactive PPD when due to tuberculosis
What pathogen causes a disease characterized by acute pharyngitis and cervical lymphadenitis and is thought to have a role in the development of Burkitt lymphoma and nasopharyngeal carcinoma?	Epstein-Barr virus
What are some examples of benign neoplasms that occur in the neck?	Lipomas, hemangiomas, neuromas, and fibromas

Lymphadenopathy in the neck region may signify malignancy. What is significant about lymphadenopathy in the supraclavicular fossa?

The patient may have malignancy somewhere below the neck region (GI tract, lungs, reproductive system, kidneys).

When the cause of a neck mass is unclear, in general, what is the best imaging modality for evaluating it?

CT with contrast

CHAPTER 15

Chest Pain and Palpitations

CHEST PAIN

What conditions can cause cardiovascular chest pain?	Coronary artery disease, aortic dissection, pericarditis, myocarditis, valvular heart disease
What conditions can cause musculoskeletal chest pain?	Costochondritis, rheumatoid arthritis, fibromyalgia, psoriatic arthritis, fractures, osteomyelitis, septic arthritis, sickle cell disease
What conditions can cause pulmonary chest pain?	Pulmonary embolism, pleurisy, pneumothorax, pneumonia
What are other causes of chest pain?	Anxiety, herpes zoster, gastroesophageal disease

COSTOCHONDRITIS

What are the clinical manifestations of costochondritis?	Sharp pain that localizes to a specific area, pain that lasts for hours to weeks, pain worse with deep breathing, chest wall tenderness to palpation
Does tenderness to palpation rule out nonmusculoskeletal diseases?	No. Musculoskeletal diseases can coexist with life-threatening conditions.

What is the management of costochondritis?	Avoid any activity that exacerbates the pain, topical pain medication (capsaicin, salicylate, nonsteroidal anti-inflammatories), oral nonsteroidal anti-inflammatories
How long does costochondritis typically last?	2-4 weeks

CORONARY ARTERY DISEASE

Describe the initial pathogenesis of atherosclerosis.	Endothelial injury leads to increased leukocyte adhesion to the endothelium, increased endothelial permeability, and endothelial release of hemostatic and vasoactive substances.
How is angina pectoris diagnosed?	Clinical history of a retrosternal pressure-like or squeezing sensation, frequently with radiation to the arms, neck, and jaw
Chest pain relief with nitroglycerin is diagnostic for angina. True or false?	False. Nitroglycerin can also decrease pain due to esophageal spasm.
What characterizes chronic stable angina?	Reproducibility with a consistent amount of exertion and long-standing symptoms
How is exercise-induced angina diagnosed?	Stress test results demonstrate ST depression during exercise.
Which stress-test findings may imply a poorer prognosis in cases of chronic stable angina?	ST depression greater than 2 mm, ischemia at low stress levels, hypotension resulting from exertion, the presence of ischemic changes in more than five EKG leads
What three general management strategies should be considered in chronic stable angina?	1. Modification of risk factors 2. Symptomatic relief of angina via medication or interventional modalities 3. Treatment of other contributing diseases

What other diseases may exacerbate chronic stable angina?

Fever, anemia, congestive heart failure, infection, thyrotoxicosis

What medications may provide symptomatic relief of angina?

Nitrates, calcium channel blockers, beta-blockers

Describe the mechanism by which nitrates provide symptomatic relief.

Vasodilation of the following:

Coronary vessels → increase myocardial oxygen supply

Peripheral veins → decrease venous return to the heart → preload reduction → decrease in myocardial oxygen demand

Peripheral arteries → decrease in peripheral vascular resistance → afterload reduction → decrease in myocardial oxygen demand

Do nitrates have a predominant effect on veins or arteries?

Veins (and therefore preload)

Describe the mechanism by which beta-blockers and calcium channel blockers provide symptomatic relief.

Decrease myocardial oxygen demand by decreasing heart rate (HR), blood pressure (BP), and contractility

If angina continues despite maximal medical management, what strategies may be employed?

Cardiac catheterization to evaluate coronary anatomy; revascularization can be considered via coronary angioplasty, stenting, or CABG

Describe Prinzmetal variant angina.

Angina at rest characterized by transient coronary artery spasm and ST elevation

What conditions fall under the heading of acute coronary syndromes (ACS)?

Unstable angina (UA), non-ST-elevation myocardial infarction (MI) (NSTEMI), ST-elevation MI (STEMI)

What physical exam findings are typical of ACS?

Tachycardia, transient S3 or S4, hypertension, mitral regurgitation secondary to ischemia of the papillary muscle

Describe UA.

New onset angina (<2 months) with only minimal exertion, crescendo angina in the setting of existing stable angina, angina at rest of greater than 20 minutes, angina occurring greater than 24 hours post-MI

What EKG findings may be seen in UA?

ST depression or symmetric T-wave inversions

In what percentage of patients does UA progress to MI?

Approximately 5%

In cases of UA, what are the major steps for providing symptomatic relief and preserving myocardial function?

Provide analgesia, improve coronary blood flow, prevent coronary thrombosis, decrease myocardial oxygen demand

What drug options should be considered to address analgesia?

Morphine to decrease pain and anxiety

Why is it important to control pain in a patient with UA?

Analgesia can decrease the sympathetic response (lower HR and BP), which decreases myocardial oxygen demand.

When should antiplatelet therapy be started?

Immediately after UA is suspected

What drug should be used to provide antiplatelet action acutely?

Aspirin 162-325 mg

What drug options should be used to provide long-term antiplatelet action?

Aspirin 81-325 mg and clopidogrel 75 mg, daily

What class of drugs should be used to reduce myocardial demand in all patients with UA/NSTEMI?

Beta-blockers

Is thrombolytic therapy used in the treatment of UA and NSTEMI?

No

Following stabilization of the UA/NSTEMI patient, what further studies should be undertaken in low-risk patients?

Noninvasive stress testing

In high-risk patients?

Cardiac catheterization followed by revascularization procedures, if indicated

How is UA differentiated from NSTEMI?

In NSTEMI, ischemia is significant enough to cause myocardial damage, leading to an elevation of troponin I and creatine kinase from cardiac muscle (CK-MB)

| Which biomarker is the most sensitive and specific for myocardial injury? | Troponin I |

| How are NSTEMI and STEMI similar? | In both conditions, troponin I and CK-MB are elevated. |

| How are NSTEMI and STEMI different? | In STEMIs, EKGs show ST segment elevations or Q waves in at least two contiguous leads. In NSTEMIs, EKGs show ST segment depression but lack ST segment elevations or Q waves. |

EKG changes in which leads are indicative of

Anterior wall ischemia?	V1-V6
Anteroseptal ischemia?	V1-V3
Lateral ischemia?	AVL, I, V4-V6
Inferior ischemia?	II, III, aVF

| What group of patients are more likely to present with atypical symptoms of myocardial infarction? | Women, diabetics, the elderly |

| What accounts for most of the deaths that take place within a few hours of a STEMI? | Ventricular tachyarrhythmia |

| Describe the time-course of EKG changes in a STEMI. | Refer to the table below: |

EKG Changes during a STEMI

Immediate	Minutes	Hours	24-48 Hours	Day-Weeks
Hyperacute T waves	ST elevation	Q-wave, T-wave inversion	ST back to baseline	T-wave normalizes

What does echocardiography show during STEMI?

LV hypokinesis or akinesis in the area supplied by the occluded vessel

What two pharmacologic agents should be started immediately after diagnosing a patient with either NSTEMI or STEMI?

1. Aspirin
2. Anti-thrombotic agents (unfractionated or LMW heparin)

Despite its increased effectiveness, when is *LMW* heparin contraindicated?

Renal insufficiency as it is cleared by the kidneys

What further immediate steps should be taken?

MONA (morphine, oxygen, nitroglycerin, and aspirin), anxiolytics, beta-blockers

How should the first dose of aspirin be taken?

Chewed, to ensure rapid uptake

If the patient continues to show ST-elevation and has persistent angina, what therapy should be initiated?

Reperfusion with primary angioplasty or initiation of thrombolysis

Tissue plasminogen activator (tPA) can restore patency to an occluded coronary vessel in what percentage of patients?

Approximately 75%-80%

Primary angioplasty can restore patency to an occluded coronary vessel in what percentage of patients?

Approximately 95%

Beyond what period of time from the onset of initial symptoms does thrombolysis lose effectiveness?

6 hours

What is the major limitation of primary angioplasty in this clinical setting?

Lack of widespread availability

Following thrombolysis, for how long should heparin be continued?

24-48 hours

How long should aspirin be continued?

Indefinitely

What other drugs should be initiated on a long-term basis?

Beta-blockers, ACEI, high-dose statins (eg, atorvastatin 80 mg once daily)

What diagnostic study should be performed several days after acute MI?	Echocardiography
What vaccinations should be given to patients with coronary artery disease?	Annual influenza, pneumococcal

AORTIC DISSECTION

What is the pathophysiology of aortic dissection?	A tear in the intima causes the intima to separate from the media and/or adventita.
What are the risk factors for aortic dissection?	Hypertension, atherosclerosis, preexisting aortic aneurysm, vasculitis, collagen vascular disorders, family history of dissection, bicuspid aortic valve, aortic coarctation, Turner syndrome, coronary artery bypass graft surgery, previous aortic valve replacement, cardiac catheterization, trauma, cocaine use
What trauma classically can cause dissection?	Rapid deceleration from a motor vehicle accident
What are the clinical manifestations of aortic dissection?	Sharp, tearing chest or back pain; weak or absent carotid, brachial, or femoral pulses; more than 20 mm Hg difference in systolic BP between the right and left arms
What are the complications of aortic dissection?	Aortic insufficiency, myocardial infarction, tamponade, hemothorax, stroke, Horner syndrome (from compression of the cervical sympathetic ganglion), vocal cord paralysis (from compression of the left recurrent laryngeal nerve)
What imaging findings can be seen with aortic dissection?	Mediastinal widening on chest x-ray, two distinct aortic lumens and an intimal flap on chest CT scan with intravenous (IV) contrast or MRI, transesophageal echocardiogram confirming a true and false lumen
What is the management of aortic dissection involving the ascending aorta?	Emergent surgery due to high risk for complications (the mortality rate is 1%-2% per hour)

What is the management of aortic dissection involving the descending aorta?	IV beta-blockers to reduce heart rate and BP (and, thus, vascular stress)

VALVULAR DISEASE

Besides mitral regurgitation, what is the most common cause of valvular disease?	Aortic stenosis (AS)
What is a normal aortic valve area?	3-4 cm^2 in adults
What is the aortic valve area in critical AS?	Less than 0.8 cm^2
List the three most common causes of AS.	1. Bicuspid aortic valve 2. Degenerative changes associated with the aging process (primarily sclerosis) 3. Rheumatic fever
What are the symptoms of AS?	Angina, CHF symptoms, syncope
Describe common signs in AS.	Normal to low BP, "parvus et tardus" (a weak and slow carotid pulse that often rises slowly and with a shudder), crescendo-decrescendo murmur at the right second intercostal space that typically radiates to the neck
How should AS be treated if it is asymptomatic?	No intervention is indicated.
How should the disease be managed once symptoms begin?	Surgery

PERICARDITIS

What conditions can cause pericarditis?	Viral infection (coxsackie A and B, echovirus, cytomegalovirus, human immunodeficiency virus), bacterial infection (staphylococcus, tuberculosis), post MI, cardiac surgery or procedures, chest trauma, uremia, dialysis, hypothyroidism, radiation, malignancy (lung, breast, Hodgkin), collagen vascular disease, idiopathic

What are the clinical manifestations of pericarditis?

Pleuritic chest pain (relieved by leaning forward), pericardial friction rub (scratchy sound heard best with the diaphragm of the stethoscope at the left sternal border), diffuse concave upward ST elevation

Why are echocardiograms ordered for pericarditis?

To evaluate for pericardial effusions and tamponade (if suspected)

What is the treatment for idiopathic or viral pericarditis?

Nonsteroidal anti-inflammatories (eg, ibuprofen) or aspirin

VENOUS THROMBOEMBOLISM

What are the three factors typically involved in thrombosis formation (and also make up Virchow triad)?

1. Stasis of blood flow
2. Vascular endothelial injury
3. Hypercoagulable state

What is Homans sign?

Calf pain with passive ankle dorsiflexion associated with the presence of a deep venous thrombosis (DVT) (a frequently pimped but unreliable examination finding)

What physical examination findings suggest a DVT?

Local edema (>3-cm diameter increase compared to the unaffected side), pain, warmth, a palpable cord (indicating a thrombosed vein), presence of newly developed varicose veins

What is the imaging study of choice to rule out DVT?

Compression ultrasonography

What is the role of D-dimers in the workup of suspected DVT?

D-dimer levels <500 ng/mL are helpful in excluding DVTs.

What are the risk factors for thrombosis?

Refer to the table on next page:

Inherited and Acquired Risk Factors for Thrombosis

	Risk Factor	Mechanism/Comments
Inherited	Protein C (PC) deficiency	PC inactivates coagulation factors (CF) 5a and 8a
	Factor 5 Leiden mutation	• With the mutation, factor 5 is resistant to protein C inactivation • The most common inherited cause
	Prothrombin (aka CF 2) gene mutation	The mutation increases CF 2 synthesis
	Antithrombin deficiency	
	Protein S (PS) deficiency	The action of PC is dependent on PS
Acquired	Malignancy	• Increased production of procoagulants • Check stool for occult blood (colorectal cancer) • Rectal exam in males (prostate cancer) • Pelvic exam in females
	Trauma	
	Pregnancy	Increased stasis from uterine obstruction of venous return and increased PC resistance
	Drugs	Eg, oral contraceptive pills, hormone replacement therapy, and tamoxifen
	Immobilization	
	Heart failure	
	Hyperhomocysteinemia	
	Antiphospholipid antibodies	• *In vitro* increase in a PTT that does not correct with mixing • Ask about prior fetal loss • Ask about meds (hydralazine, procainamide, and phenothiazines)
	Myeloproliferative disorders	Eg, essential thrombocythemia and polycythemia vera
	Hyperviscosity syndromes	Eg, Waldenstrom macroglobulinemia and multiple myeloma
	Recent surgery	Especially orthopedic surgeries
	Nephrotic syndrome	Loss of antithrombin, PC, and PS
	Obesity	
	Prior venous thromboembolism	

Do all DVT patients need a workup for an inherited thrombophilia?

No

What is the management of a DVT?

Unfractionated or low-molecular-weight heparin (LMWH) and warfarin

For how many days should treatment with heparin and warfarin overlap?

At least 4-5 days

If heparin and warfarin have overlapped sufficiently and international normalized ratio (INR) has been therapeutic for two consecutive days, what should you do?

Discontinue heparin and continue warfarin alone.

How long should you continue oral anticoagulation with warfarin in the following scenarios?

The cause of the venous thromboembolism (VTE) is reversible

3 months

It is the patient's first idiopathic VTE

6-12 months

The cause of the VTE is irreversible or if the patient has cancer

Indefinitely

What does INR stand for?

International normalized ratio

By whom and why was it developed?

By the World Health Organization (WHO) in order to standardize prothrombin times

What INR is considered therapeutic for warfarin treatment of DVTs?

2-3

What should be done if anticoagulation is contraindicated (eg, active bleeding) or if anticoagulation has failed?

Place an inferior vena cava (IVC) filter

Is LMWH at least as effective as unfractionated heparin?

Yes

What are the advantages of using LMWH versus unfractionated heparin?

Longer half-life allows for once or twice daily dosing, doses are fixed, monitoring of the activated partial thromboplastin time (aPTT) is not required, thrombocytopenia is less likely

What percentage of symptomatic, untreated, proximal DVT patients will develop pulmonary embolism?	50%
What are the symptoms associated with pulmonary embolism (PE)?	Dyspnea, pleuritic pain, cough, hemoptysis
What are the signs associated with PE?	Tachypnea, rales, diaphoresis, tachycardia, heart gallop, a loud second heart sound
What chest x-ray (CXR) findings suggest a PE?	Atelectasis, Hampton hump, Westermark sign
What is Hampton hump on CXR?	A triangular pleural-based density with an apex that points toward the hilum
What is Westermark sign?	Oligemia distal to the infarction
Although the EKG is often normal, a PE may cause what EKG changes?	Sinus tachycardia, right bundle branch block, $S_I Q_{III} T_{III}$
What is $S_I Q_{III} T_{III}$?	Prominent S wave in lead I, Q wave in III, T-wave inversion in III
What arterial blood gas findings suggest PE?	Hypoxemia, hypocapnia, respiratory alkalosis
What other diagnostic studies are used in suspected PE?	D-dimer, ventilation/perfusion (V/Q) scan, spiral CT, pulmonary angiography

PNEUMOTHORAX

What is a primary pneumothorax?	A pneumothorax without a precipitating event in patients who do not have lung disease
What is the pathophysiology of a primary pneumothorax?	Rupture of a subpleural bleb
What are risk factors for primary pneumothoraces?	Smoking, family history, Marfan syndrome, homocystinuria, thoracic endometriosis

What are the clinical manifestations of a pneumothorax?	Sudden onset of dyspnea and pleuritic chest pain, diminished breath sounds on the affected side, hyperresonance to percussion, subcutaneous emphysema, hypoxemia
What findings on chest x-ray are indicative of a pneumothorax?	White visceral pleural line, lack of pulmonary vascular markings beyond the visceral pleural edge
What is the treatment for a stable patient with a small pneumothorax (<2-3 cm between the lung and the chest wall on chest x-ray)?	Supplemental oxygen
What is the treatment for a larger pneumothorax?	Needle aspiration or chest tube insertion

ESOPHAGEAL CAUSES OF CHEST PAIN

What percentage of patients with recurrent noncardiac chest pain have gastroesophageal reflux?	50%
How should patients with noncardiac chest pain and suspected gastroesophageal reflux be managed?	Meta analyses have indicated that a clinical response to an empiric trial of a proton pump inhibitor (twice daily for 8 weeks) performs well as a diagnostic test compared to esophageal pH testing.

PALPITATIONS

What are palpitations?	An unpleasant awareness of a forceful, rapid, or irregular heart beat
What are psychiatric causes of palpitations?	Panic disorder, generalized anxiety disorder, somatization, depression
What are cardiac causes of palpitations?	Supraventricular tachycardia, ventricular ectopy, nonsustained ventricular tachycardia, atrial fibrillation, atrial flutter, tachycardia with variable block, valvular disease, cardiomyopathy, atrial myxoma

What drugs are associated with palpitations?	Sympathomimetics, vasodilators (which can cause reflex tachycardia), anticholinergics, cocaine, nicotine, caffeine
What are other causes of palpitations?	Hypoglycemia, thyrotoxicosis, pheochromocytoma
What test should be performed for all patients with palpitations?	EKG
How do Holter monitors differ from continuous loop event recorders?	Holter monitors save data for 24-48 hours with patients keeping a log of symptoms. Event recorders only save data preceding and following an event (patients manually activate the monitor).
Which has a higher diagnostic yield for palpitations?	Continuous loop event recorders

ATRIAL FIBRILLATION

Define the following types of atrial fibrillation.	
Paroxysmal	Episode terminates spontaneously in less than 7 days
Persistent	Episode fails to resolve within 7 days
Permanent	Episode lasts for more than 1 year
Lone	Paroxysmal, persistent, or permanent atrial fibrillation in patients without structural heart disease
What is the rhythm in atrial fibrillation?	Irregularly irregular
What diagnostic tests should be obtained in atrial fibrillation?	EKG, echocardiogram, thyroid stimulating hormone (to evaluate for thyrotoxicosis)

What is the utility of echocardiogram in atrial fibrillation?

Evaluate for structural heart disease; patients with left atrial enlargement (>4 cm) are unlikely to remain in normal sinus rhythm if cardioverted; transesophageal echocardiograms can evaluate for left atrial or left atrial appendage thrombi, suggesting that the patient does not need four weeks of warfarin and can be cardioverted.

What are the management decisions in atrial fibrillation?

Rate control with beta-blockers or calcium channel blockers versus rhythm control with electric or pharmacologic cardioversion, anticoagulation to prevent emboli

What did the Atrial Fibrillation Follow-up Investigation of Rhythm Management (AFFIRM) trial indicate?

The AFFIRM trial indicated that rhythm control does not decrease the rate of embolic events compared to rate control.

In the absence of anticoagulation, what percentage of patients with atrial fibrillation will have a stroke each year?

3%-5%

What score can be used to predict the annual risk of stroke in patients with atrial fibrillation?

CHADS2 score

How is the CHADS2 score calculated?

Congestive heart failure (1 point), hypertension (1 point), age ≥75 (1 point), diabetes mellitus (1 point), prior stroke (2 points)

Which patients should receive anticoagulation with warfarin (INR target 2-3)?

Patients with CHADS2 scores of 2 or more

What is the treatment for patients with CHADS2 scores of 1?

Aspirin or warfarin

What is the treatment for patients with a CHADS2 score of 0?

Aspirin 325 mg once daily

ELECTROCARDIOGRAPHY

On an electrocardiography (EKG),
what is

The unit of measurement on the x axis?	Seconds
The unit of measurement on the y axis?	Millivolts
The dimensions of a small box?	1 × 1 mm
The dimensions of a large box?	5 × 5 mm
The length of time represented by a small box?	0.04 seconds
The length of time represented by a large box?	0.2 seconds (or 0.04 seconds × 5)
The name for a positive or negative deflection from the baseline?	Wave
The name for a line between two waves?	Segment
The name for a segment and wave combination?	Interval
Where are the precordial leads placed?	V1: 4th intercostal space (ICS), to the right of the sternum; V2: 4th ICS, to the left of the sternum; V3: between V2 and V4; V4: 5th ICS, at the mid-clavicular line; V5: at the same level as V4 at the anterior axillary line; V6: at the same level as V4 and V5, at the mid-axillary line
What represents atrial contraction?	P wave
What represents ventricular contraction?	QRS complex
What represents ventricular repolarization?	T wave
When reading an EKG, what components should be covered?	Rate, rhythm, axis, intervals, hypertrophy, evidence of myocardial infarction

How can the rate be determined?

Here are two ways: (1) Count the number of big boxes between QRS complexes. 1 big box = 300 beats per minute (bpm); 2 = 150 bpm; 3 = 100 bpm; 4 = 75 bpm; 5 = 60 bpm; 6 = 50 bpm. It's helpful to memorize the sequence: 300-150-100-75-60-50. (2) Count the number of QRS complexes on the last line at the bottom of the page and multiply that number by 6 (the rhythm strip represents 10 seconds worth of electrical activity).

What does normal sinus rhythm (NSR) indicate?

NSR indicates that the electrical impulse in the heart is generated by the sinoatrial node and is following the heart's normal circuitry (ie, from the sinoatrial node to the atrioventricular node to the bundle of His and to the Purkinje fibers)

What EKG features indicate that the patient is in sinus rhythm and that the impulse is being generated by the sinoatrial node?

Each QRS complex is preceded by a P wave. The P waves are positive in I, II, and aVF (a positive deflection indicates that an impulse is approaching a lead. I, II, and aVF are at the inferior-lateral border of the heart, so positive P waves in these leads suggest that the impulse was generated from the sinoatrial node).

Name these rhythms.

Sinus rhythm with the rate between 60 and 100

Normal sinus rhythm

Sinus rhythm with the rate greater than 100

Sinus tachycardia

Sinus rhythm with the rate less than 60

Sinus bradycardia

What does the axis represent?

The mean QRS vector—this is the summation of the amplitude and directionality of all the small vectors that make up ventricular depolarization. Since the left ventricle dominates ventricular depolarization, the mean QRS vector normally points inferiorly and to the patient's left.

Which leads are used to determine axis?

First look at the QRS complexes in leads I and aVF. If the QRS complex is positive in lead I and negative in aVF, look at lead II.

What is the axis?

QRS complex is positive in lead I and aVF

Normal

QRS complex is positive in lead I, negative in aVF, and positive in lead II

Normal

QRS complex is positive in lead I, negative in aVF, and negative in lead II

Left-axis deviation

QRS complex is negative in lead I and positive in aVF

Right-axis deviation

QRS complex is negative in lead I and aVF

Northwest axis (also called extreme right axis deviation or indeterminate)

What is a normal PR interval?

Between 0.12 seconds (three small boxes) and 0.2 seconds (five small boxes)

What is the normal duration for a QRS complex?

Less than 0.12 seconds (three small boxes)

What is the equation for calculating the correct QT interval?

QTc = QT interval/square root of the RR interval (in seconds)

Why is the QT interval corrected?

The QT interval represents ventricular repolarization, which is dependent on the heart rate. With faster heart rates, the QT interval is shorter (and vice versa for slower heart rates).

What constitutes a prolonged QTc interval?

Greater than 0.44 seconds

What EKG changes can be seen in a myocardial infarction (MI)?

ST segment elevation (although ST segment depression can be seen in non-ST elevation MIs); T-wave inversion; Q waves (must be in at least two contiguous leads)

Which areas of the heart correspond to EKG changes in these leads?

II, III, aVF

Inferior: typically supplied by either the right coronary or circumflex arteries

V1-V6

Anterior: supplied by the left anterior descending artery

I, aVL, V5, V6

Lateral: supplied by the circumflex artery

CHAPTER 16

Cough

AIRWAY INFECTIONS

What is bronchiolitis?

An airway disease (usually viral lower respiratory tract infection) characterized by acute inflammation, edema, and necrosis of the bronchiolar walls; hypersecretion of mucus; and bronchospasm

In what patient population is bronchiolitis most common?

Infants

What is the most common etiology of bronchiolitis?

Respiratory syncytial virus (RSV)

Does infection with RSV confer immunity?

No. Reinfection can occur.

What is the name of the vaccine used to help prevent RSV infection (routinely given to infants with a history of chronic lung or heart disease or prematurity)?

Palivizumab

How is a diagnosis of bronchiolitis made?

It is a clinical diagnosis. An upper respiratory infection developing into a lower respiratory infection with signs of respiratory distress including wheezing, tachypnea, and increased work of breathing (nasal flaring, grunting, retractions).

What is ribavirin?

An antiviral used to treat severe bronchiolitis (or those at risk for severe disease)

What is acute bronchitis?

Transient inflammation of the bronchi (medium and large airways)

What are the causes of acute bronchitis?

Viruses (most often), bacterial, inhalation of foreign material (toxic fumes, etc)

What age group is most commonly affected by acute bronchitis?

Children less than 5 years old

What are the signs and symptoms of acute bronchitis due to infection?

Fever, cough and sputum production, shortness of breath, wheezing, chest pain, and/or malaise

How long does acute bronchitis usually last?

20-30 days

What is the treatment of acute bronchitis?

Rest and plenty of fluids, acetaminophen or other pain relievers, cough drops, expectorant cough medication (eg, guaifenesin), cough suppressants for nonproductive cough (eg, dextromethorphan), bronchodilators, antibiotics (only when bacterial cause suspected or if patient has chronic lung disease)

The American Academy of Pediatrics strongly recommends that cough and cold medications not be given to children younger than what age because of life-threatening side effects?

2 years old

Evidence shows that cough and cold medicines are not effective in children younger than what age?

6 years old

What can caregivers give children to reduce coughing?

A small amount of honey may be given to children over 1 year old. Throat lozenges or cough drops may be given to children over 4 years old.

What is croup?

Common infection that causes acute inflammation of trachea and larynx

What is the most common cause?

Parainfluenza virus

What symptoms are seen with croup?

Hoarseness, barking cough

In what age group does croup occur?

Children 6 months to 12 years, most commonly in children 1-3 years of age

What is the radiographic finding known as the "steeple sign?"

Anteroposterior (AP) view of the neck shows narrowing trachea.

What is the treatment?

Steroids, nebulizer treatments, cool humidified air, racemic epinephrine

What is the infectious agent of pertussis (whooping cough)?	*Bordetella pertussis*
What are the classic symptoms?	Whooping cough spells (paroxysms) followed by posttussive emesis
What are the three stages of disease?	1. Catarrhal stage (mild upper respiratory infection symptoms) 2. Paroxysmal (whooping cough) 3. Convalescent (mild cough continues)
How long may it last?	12 weeks
Do antibiotics abort the disease?	Only in the catarrhal phase
What is the main purpose of antibiotics in this setting?	To decrease spread to others
What is the treatment of choice?	Erythromycin for 14 days for patient and close contacts
What is the concerning possible complication of erythromycin in infants?	Hypertrophic pyloric stenosis
What are alternatives to erythromycin?	Other macrolides (eg, azithromycin)

PNEUMONITIS

What is pneumonitis?	Inflammation of the lung parenchyma
What is pneumonia?	Pneumonitis due to infection
What are some common symptoms of pneumonia?	Rigors, fatigue, cough (may be dry or productive), sputum production, pleuritic chest pain, dyspnea
What are the common physical signs of pneumonia?	Fever, tachypnea, dullness to chest percussion, tactile fremitus, egophony, bronchial breath sounds, crackles or rales to auscultation
What is the pneumonia severity index?	A prognostic model that is used to help determine whether a patient with pneumonia should be treated as an inpatient or outpatient
What are the CURB-65 criteria?	It is a clinical prediction rule that uses risk factors (confusion, uremia, respiratory rate >30, BP <90/60 mm Hg, and age over 65) to predict mortality and need for hospitalization in pneumonia. 0-1 factors treat as an outpatient, >2 factors consider hospitalization.

Is a positive sputum culture necessary to make the diagnosis of pneumonia?

No

Clinical suspicion plus what diagnostic test result is necessary for a diagnosis of pneumonia?

Pulmonary infiltrate on chest radiograph (obtain two views)

What purpose do radiographic studies serve in the management of pneumonia?

Qualify pneumonia based on location (usually singular lobar consolidation but can be multilobar or diffuse) and possible complications (eg, pleural effusion, pneumothorax, empyema, abscess)

A chest radiograph can be negative early in the disease course of pneumonia. True or false?

True

What is community acquired pneumonia (CAP)?

Pneumonia that is not acquired in hospital or long-term care facility

What is/are the first-line antibiotic(s) for CAP in the outpatient setting when no comorbidities are present, the patient has not been on antibiotics within the last 3 months, and there is a low local prevalence of drug-resistant strains?

Macrolides (azithromycin, clarithromycin, or erythromycin) are strongly recommended. Doxycycline is an alternative.

What is/are the first-line antibiotic(s) for CAP in the outpatient setting when comorbidities (eg, heart/lung/liver/renal disease, diabetes, malignancy, alcoholism, asplenia, immune deficiency) are present and/or the patient has been on antibiotics within the last 3 months and/or there is a high risk of drug-resistance?

A fluoroquinolone or macrolide plus β-lactum

What is the minimum duration of antibiotic therapy for uncomplicated CAP?

5 days (assuming the patient is stable and has been afebrile for more than 48 hours)

What is the most common bacterial cause of CAP in adults?

Streptococcus pneumoniae

What additional etiologies of pneumonia should you keep in mind for a patient with a history of the following:

COPD and/or smoking

Haemophilus influenzae, Pseudomonas aeruginosa, Legionella, Moraxella catarrhalis

Immune suppression

H. influenzae, Pneumocystis jirovecii, Cryptococcus, Histoplasma, Aspergillus, P. aeruginosa, Mycobacterium tuberculosis, atypical mycobacteria

Seizures

Aspiration: oral anaerobes, gram-negative enteric pathogens, *Staphylococcus aureus*

Alcoholism

Aspiration, *Klebsiella, Acinetobacter, M. tuberculosis*

Recent animal exposure

Francisella tularensis (deer, rabbits); Hantavirus, Yersinia pestis (rodents); *Histoplasma capsulatum* (bat and bird droppings); Q fever, Brucellosis (some farm animals); H5N1 virus (poultry)

Residence or travel to the Southwest United States

Coccidioides species, *Hantavirus*

What patients are particularly prone to infection with *S. pneumoniae*?

Those with history of splenectomy, sickle cell disease, lung disease, HIV, and/or renal failure

What are the most common causes of pneumonia in young, healthy adults?

Mycoplasma, Chlamydia, viruses

What is pneumonia due to these organisms called?

Atypical pneumonia

Is the disease more or less severe than typical pneumonia?

Generally the illness is mild.

Do chest x-rays correlate well with the degree of illness in atypical pneumonia?

No. Chest x-rays often appear disproportionately "worse than the patient."

What are the most common causes of pneumonia in young children?

Respiratory viruses (respiratory syncytial virus [RSV], parainfluenza, adenovirus, enterovirus)

What are some common causes of bacterial pneumonia in children?

S. pneumoniae, group A *Streptococcus,* group B *Streptococcus* (in a neonate), *M. pneumoniae, Chlamydia trachomatis, H. influenzae, M. catarrhalis*

What is the treatment for pneumonia due to influenza A?

Give oseltamivir or zanamivir within 48 hours of symptom onset. Consider empirical antibiotics for secondary bacterial pneumonia (*S. aureus, S. pneumoniae*).

What are the risk factors for developing pneumonia due to *S. aureus*?

Viral pneumonia (eg, influenza), infection via hematogenous route (ie, IV drug users or patients with infective endocarditis), diabetes, liver disease

Urinary antigen test exists for what pathogens?

Legionella and *S. pneumoniae*

What is the major water source for *Legionella*?

Water distribution systems of large buildings (eg, hotels, hospitals)

What populations are most susceptible to *Legionella* pneumonia?

Elderly, smokers, immunocompromised, travelers

What symptoms are common in a patient with *Legionella* pneumonia?

Dry cough, fever, headache, confusion, weakness, GI disturbances (diarrhea)

What is the typical description for the sputum in *Klebsiella* infection?

Currant jelly sputum

Patients with what underlying diseases are at increased risk for *Pseudomonas* pneumonia?

Patients with diabetes or cystic fibrosis

What is the most common opportunistic infection in HIV patients?

Pneumocystis pneumonia (PCP) caused by *P. jirovecii*

What is the treatment for PCP?

Trimethoprim-sulfamethoxazole and steroids

What is the most common cause of pneumonia in an HIV patient?

S. pneumoniae (same as in the immunocompetent population)

What causes chemical pneumonitis?

Aspiration of sterile gastric contents

What are the typical signs and symptoms of chemical pneumonitis?

Dyspnea, cough, low-grade fever, infiltrates on CXR involving dependent areas of lung

LUNG CANCER

What is the leading cause of cancer deaths in both men and women?	Lung cancer
What is the most prominent risk factor for developing lung cancer?	Smoking, including exposure to second-hand smoking
Which types of lung cancer are typically located centrally?	Small cell and squamous cell
Which lung cancer is not linked to smoking and is more common in women?	Bronchoalveolar adenocarcinoma
What is the most common symptom of lung cancer?	Chronic cough
What are some other causes of chronic cough (lasts more than 8 weeks)?	Tobacco smoking, chronic exposure to environmental irritants, postnasal drip (allergic rhinitis, chronic sinusitis), medication (ACE inhibitors), asthma, COPD, gastroesophageal reflux disease, infection (tuberculosis)
What are other signs and symptoms of lung cancer?	Hemoptysis, stridor, dyspnea, hoarseness, dysphagia, associated paraneoplastic syndromes
What is a Pancoast tumor?	It is a tumor of the pulmonary apex and can cause SVC syndrome and Horner syndrome.
What is superior vena cava (SVC) syndrome?	A tumor obstructs venous blood flow in the SVC causing facial swelling, headaches, and dyspnea
What typically worsens the symptoms of a patient with SVC?	Lying down or sleeping
What are the three signs typical of Horner syndrome?	1. Ptosis 2. Miosis 3. Anhidrosis
With which type of lung cancer do you more often see hypercalcemia?	Squamous cell lung cancer due to its association with parathyroid hormone-related protein (PTHrp)

With which type of lung cancer do you more often have problems with hyponatremia?

Small cell lung cancer due to association with syndrome of inappropriate antidiuretic hormone (SIADH)

How is lung cancer diagnosed?

Through imaging with CXR and CT, but biopsy gives the definitive diagnosis

Inhalation of what type of fiber may cause mesothelioma (cancer of the mesothelial lining of the lung)?

Asbestos

CHAPTER 17

Joint and Muscle Pain

SYNOVITIS AND TENOSYNOVITIS

What is synovitis?

Inflammation of the synovial lining of a joint; can be seen in gout, rheumatoid arthritis, lupus, and other inflammatory conditions

What is tenosynovitis?

Inflammation of the fluid-filled sheath, the synovium, surrounding a tendon

What are the Kanavel signs for tenosynovitis in a digit?

STEP
Symmetric swelling
Tenderness limited to the flexor sheath
Extension painful
Posture flexed

What is the mechanism of injury for many cases of septic tenosynovitis?

Penetrating trauma or puncture wound, often from dog bite

If you suspect a septic tenosynovitis, what should you do?

Parenteral antibiotics with coverage for *Staphylococcus* and *Streptococcus* and reevaluate in 12 hours; oral antibiotics for 7-14 days, total

If a patient with tenosynovitis does not respond to initial antibiotics, or if infection is purulent, what is the next step?

Urgent evaluation for surgical drainage

DEGENERATIVE JOINT DISEASE

What is the most common joint disorder?

Osteoarthritis (OA)

Describe the pathogenesis of OA.	Progressive destruction of articular cartilage by proteolytic enzymes, remodeling of subchondral bone
What are the most common joints involved in localized idiopathic OA?	Weight bearing (knees, hips, and cervical and lumbar spine), hands (distal interphalangeals [DIPs], distal interphalangeals [PIPs], carpal metacarpals [CMCs]), feet (metatarsal phalangeals [MTPs])
What spinal levels are most commonly involved?	C5; T8; L3: areas of greatest flexibility
At least how many joints must be involved for generalized idiopathic OA?	Three
What are the risk factors associated with idiopathic OA?	Advanced age, female sex, obesity
What are some predisposing factors of secondary OA?	Repeated joint stress, genetic collagen abnormalities, metabolic and endocrine diseases (hemochromatosis, diabetes mellitus, hypothyroidism), inflammatory joint diseases, neuropathic arthropathy
What is the most common symptom of OA?	Dull, achy pain aggravated by joint use and relieved by rest. Pain may occur at rest and at night with advanced disease. It is usually localized and asymmetrical.
What are the key physical examination findings of OA?	Heberden and Bouchard nodes, squared appearance of hand if first CMC joint involved, osteophytes, limited movement, crepitus, joint effusion, malalignment in advanced cases
What are osteophytes?	Bony enlargements at joint margins formed in response to cartilage degeneration
What joint when enlarged in OA is called a Heberden node?	DIP
What joint when enlarged in OA is called a Bouchard node?	PIP

What is the most likely result of the following laboratory tests in OA?

Rheumatoid factor

Normal, although may be elevated in elderly

ESR

Normal, except in unusual inflammatory variations

Synovial fluid

Clear color, viscous fluid, WBC count $<2000/mm^3$

What are the complications of OA in the following locations?

Feet

Hallux valgus or Hallux rigiditus at MTP

Knees

Baker cysts, varus angulation, valgus angulation

Spine

Osteophytes arising from vertebral bodies may lead to spinal cord compression/spinal stenosis, spondylolisthesis (slipping of one vertebral body on another)

What are the usual treatment options of OA in terms in each category?

Lifestyle modifications and conservative management options

Balancing rest and exercise, physical therapy, weight loss, joint protection, physiotherapy (heat, cold, ultrasound), orthotics

Pharmacologic options

Acetaminophen and/or tramadol, NSAIDs in combination with GI protecting agent (only for short-term use), intra-articular corticosteroids

Surgical options

Arthroscopic irrigation or synovectomy, arthroplasty, artificial joints

What are appropriate indications for an intra-articular corticosteroid injection?

Rheumatoid arthritis, osteoarthritis, crystal-induced arthritis, tenosynovitis and bursitis, entrapment neuropathies

What are the most common local side effects after a corticosteroid injection?

Lipodystrophy, discomfort, loss of skin pigmentation, transient increased pain for 24-48 hours

What injection sites have an increased risk of infection and should be injected judiciously when other treatment options have failed?

Olecranon and prepatellar bursae

What are some of the adverse systemic effects of corticosteroid injections?

Transient serum cortisol suppression, hyperglycemia

What are the key differences distinguishing OA from RA in terms of the following:

Refer to the table below:

	OA	RA
Stiffness	Stiffness made worse with activity and relieved with rest	Morning stiffness is significant, lasts >1 hour
Swelling of joints	Hard, bony	Soft, tender, warm
Typical finger joints involved	DIPs and CMCs of thumbs	PIPs, MCPs
X-ray findings	Asymmetric narrowing of joint space, subchondral sclerosis, marginal osteophyte formation	Erosions, cysts

RHEUMATOID ARTHRITIS

What is the pathogenesis of rheumatoid arthritis (RA)?

Autoimmune disorder involving chronic inflammation of the synovial lining of joints and destruction of the surrounding joint architecture

RA typically affects what gender and age group of patients?

Females between 30 and 55 years old

What is the typical presentation of RA?

Pain and swelling of the hands and feet, fatigue, morning stiffness

What are the most common joints involved in RA?

MCP and PIP joints of the fingers, IP joints of the thumbs, wrists, MTP joints

Is the typical joint distribution in RA symmetric or asymmetric?

Symmetric

What criteria are used in the diagnosis of RA?

Four of the following seven criteria must be satisfied for diagnosis:
1. Morning stiffness for 6 weeks
2. Arthritis of three or more joint areas simultaneously for 6 weeks
3. Arthritis of hand joints for 6 weeks
4. Symmetric arthritis
5. Rheumatoid nodules
6. Positive serum rheumatoid factor
7. Characteristic radiographic changes in the hands

How does a joint affected by RA look on x-ray?

Joint space narrowing and bony erosions

What percentage of patients with RA are RF positive?

85%

What are the classic hand deformities associated with chronic RA?

Ulnar deviation of the hands and swan neck or Boutonniere deformities of the fingers

Describe the swan neck deformity.

PIP hyperextension with distal interphalangeal (DIP) flexion

Describe the Boutonniere deformity.

PIP hyperflexion with DIP hyperextension

What are the extra-articular (systemic) manifestations of RA?

Interstitial lung disease, pericardial effusions, ocular manifestations

How is disease activity assessed in a patient with chronic RA?

Symptoms, functional status, degree of joint and extra-articular involvement, radiographic changes

What laboratory tests are used to follow the degree of synovial inflammation?

Erythrocyte sedimentation rate (ESR), C-reactive protein (CRP) levels

What is the goal of treatment of RA patients?

Early identification and treatment of active disease to prevent permanent destruction of joints

Describe the effectiveness of the five classes of drugs used for treatment of RA.

1. Analgesics

Used for pain control but no effect on disease progression

2. Nonsteroidal anti-inflammatory drugs (NSAIDs)

Have both analgesic and anti-inflammatory properties but no effect on disease outcome

3. Glucocorticoids

Effective relief of joint pain and inflammation with possible delay of joint erosions

4. Disease modifying anti-rheumatic drugs (DMARDs), for example, Methotrexate

Decreases disease activity, but limited by side effects

5. Antitumor necrosis factor alpha-antibody agents (etanercept, infliximab, adalimumab)

Powerful anti-inflammatory effects

What are the side effects of chronic glucocorticoid use?

Cushingoid features, peptic ulcers, cataracts, osteoporosis, hyperglycemia, hypertension, immunosuppression

What are the classic cushingoid features?

Truncal obesity, buffalo hump, moon face, weight gain

How much calcium and vitamin D should patients on chronic glucocorticoids take to help prevent osteoporosis?

1000-1500 mg of calcium and 400-800 IU of vitamin D daily by diet or supplementation

What is the mechanism of action of methotrexate?

Structural analogue of folic acid that competitively binds to dihydrofolate reductase, impairing DNA/RNA synthesis and decreasing cellular proliferation

What are the side effects of methotrexate use?

Hepatotoxicity, pulmonary toxicity, myelosuppression, nephrotoxicity, aphthous ulcers

If a patient is on methotrexate, how often should you check liver function tests (LFT)?

Every 4-8 weeks

If a patient is on methotrexate, how do you monitor for and help prevent myelosuppression?

Complete blood count (CBC) every 4-8 weeks and prescribe folic acid 1 mg PO daily

GOUT

What is the pathogenesis of gout?	Deposition of monosodium urate crystals in tissues or supersaturation of the extracellular fluids
What is the relationship between hyperuricemia and gout?	All patients who develop gout have hyperuricemia at some point in their disease
Will all patients with hyperuricemia develop gout?	No
What are risk factors for developing gout?	Male sex, age between 30 and 50, obesity, hypertension, alcohol use
What medications can lead to increased uric acid levels?	Thiazide diuretics, loop diuretics, aspirin
Which joint is most commonly affected in this disease?	First MTP joint (ie, podagra)
What are the symptoms of an acute gouty attack?	Intensely painful, warm, red, swollen joint that is extremely tender to the touch
What common urologic condition can someone with gout develop?	Uric acid kidney stones
Describe the time-course of an acute gouty attack.	Inflammation reaches its peak intensity within several hours, and resolves within a few days to weeks
What is the differential diagnosis of an acute gout attack?	Pseudogout, acute septic arthritis, bacterial cellulitis, traumatic injury to joint
What is the definitive diagnostic test for gout?	Aspiration of synovial fluid from the affected joint or tophaceous material and visualization of monosodium urate crystals under polarized microscopy
What do monosodium urate crystals look like under microscopy?	Needle- or rod-shaped, negatively birefringent crystals that are yellow when parallel to the axis of slow vibration

What is the first line of treatment for an acute gouty attack?	NSAIDs (eg, indomethacin) starting at a high dose, decreased as tolerated, and stopping treatment 48 hours after the attack resolves
What drug may be used for acute gout which is effective in reducing symptoms, but has limited use because it causes GI toxicity in up to 80% of patients?	Colchicine
What drugs may be used if NSAIDs or colchicine are contraindicated or ineffective?	Corticosteroids (intra-articular or systemic)
What prophylaxis is available for patients with recurrent gout?	Antihyperuricemic or uricosuric agents
What antihyperuricemic agent is commonly used and how does it work?	Allopurinol, a xanthine oxidase inhibitor; decreases the production of uric acid
What uricosuric agent is commonly used and how does it work?	Probenecid, increases the excretion of uric acid
When should you start these prophylactic medications?	AFTER an acute attack
Uric acid is a waste product from the breakdown of what organic product?	Purines
What food items are high in purines?	Organ meats (such as liver), fish (especially herring and mackerel)
What is the effect of fasting and rapid weight loss on uric acid levels?	Increases uric acid
Moderate consumption of alcohol, especially beer, as much as doubles the likelihood of developing gout. True or false?	True
What is the name for the deposition of uric acid crystals built up in the soft tissue of a gouty joint?	Gouty Tophus

MYALGIAS AND ARTHRALGIAS

A 40-year-old woman presents to your office with complaints of chronic pain and fatigue over the last year. On examination, she has multiple areas of soft tissue tenderness, but no tenderness at the joints. What is the suspected diagnosis?

Fibromyalgia syndrome (FMS)

What is the American College of Rheumatology criteria for the diagnosis of FMS?

Generalized pain for more than three months; pain on left and right sides of the body; pain above and below the waist; pain must involve the axial skeleton; Pain, not just tenderness, at 11 or more of 18 defined trigger points

How do you test the trigger points in FMS?

Digital palpation with an approximate force of 4 kg on each of 18 trigger point sites

What other symptoms do patients with FMS often describe?

Sleep disturbance, short-term memory loss, fatigue, depression and anxiety, migraine or tension headaches, substernal chest pain, paresthesias in hands and feet

What are the lifestyle changes that can help in the treatment of FMS?

Reassurance that disease is not life-threatening; stretching, exercise, and weight loss; FMS support group or visit to established FMS clinic

What medications can be used to treat FMS?

Tricyclic antidepressants, such as amitriptyline; NSAIDs for short course (no corticosteroids or narcotics); selective serotonin reuptake inhibitor (SSRI), if severe depression; topical analgesic agents applied to tender points

Pain that persists after an original injury and is out of proportion to the initial injury is characteristic of what syndrome?

Complex regional pain syndrome (CRPS)

What is the classification of CRPS?

Type 1 (reflex sympathetic dystrophy): no identifiable nerve lesion (30%)
Type 2 (causalgia): nerve lesion (70%)

Who is commonly affected by CRPS?

Women >> men, smokers, individuals between 30 and 50 years

What are some of the hallmarks of CRPS?	Allodynia, hyperpathia, hyperesthesia, sleep disturbance, pain described as "burning or throbbing"
What physical examination signs support the diagnosis of CRPS?	Swelling, hypersensitivity, contracture, overly hot or cold, atrophy of skin and soft tissue
What is the treatment of CRPS?	Physical therapy for ROM, adaptive modalities, oral medications, psychological counseling, biofeedback
What medications can help in the treatment of CRPS?	Antidepressants, anticonvulsants, calcium-channel blockers

LUPUS

What is the pathogenesis of systemic lupus erythematosus (SLE)?	Autoimmune disease in which antibodies are formed to various parts of the cell nucleus
What organ systems are most commonly affected in SLE?	Mucocutaneous (80%-90%), musculoskeletal (75%-100%), renal, neurologic, cardiovascular, respiratory systems
Which patient population does SLE most commonly affect?	Women between the ages 15 and 40 years (female to male ratio is 6-10 to 1)
What is a common initial presentation of SLE?	Constitutional symptoms (fatigue, myalgias, fever, weight changes) in combination with skin and musculoskeletal involvement
What are the diagnostic criteria for SLE?	Four of the following eleven criteria for diagnosis:

1. Malar rash (butterfly rash)
2. Discoid rash
3. Photosensitivity
4. Oral ulcers
5. Arthritis
6. Serositis
7. Renal disorder
8. Hematologic disorder
9. Immunologic disorder
10. Neurologic disorder
11. Positive antinuclear antibody (ANA)

What are the common skin manifestations in SLE?

Malar rash; discoid rash; alopecia; ulcers in the mouth, nose, or anogenital area

Name the skin manifestations seen in SLE described below.

Acute erythematous, edematous eruption over the bridge of the nose and onto the cheeks often brought on by exposure to sunlight

Malar rash (butterfly rash)

Chronic, erythematous, discrete plaques involving the face, ears, neck, and scalp; may have scaling and involve the follicles

Discoid rash

Which joints does SLE commonly affect?

Small joints of the hands (PIPs and MCPs), wrists, and knees

The World Health Organization's five-class system to determine the severity of renal disease in lupus nephritis uses what factors?

Sediment, amount of proteinuria, serum creatinine, blood pressure (BP), anti-double stranded DNA (dsDNA) status, complement levels

What lab tests are used to screen for renal involvement in SLE?

Urine dipstick, urine microscopic evaluation, plus or minus a baseline 24-hour urine analysis for protein and creatinine

What should be monitored serially to assess renal activity in SLE?

BP and urine protein

Name the following autoantibodies involved in SLE.

Present in almost 100% of people with SLE; used for diagnosis

ANA

Highly specific for SLE and associated with lupus nephritis, used to predict disease flares

Anti-dsDNA

Insensitive but highly specific for SLE diagnosis

Anti-Smith antibodies

Associated with drug-induced lupus

Antihistone antibodies

What medications can cause drug-related lupus?

Chlorpromazine, hydralazine, isoniazid, methyldopa, minocycline, procainamide, quinidine

How are the following commonly used to treat SLE?

NSAIDs	Musculoskeletal complaints
Corticosteroids	Topical for cutaneous lesions, intraarticular for joint manifestations, oral for systemic disease
Antimalarial agents, such as hydroxychloroquine	Constitutional symptoms, skin manifestations, and musculoskeletal complaints
Cyclophosphamide	Renal manifestations

What usually causes early mortality?   Renal manifestations

What usually causes late mortality?   Cardiovascular disease

CHAPTER 18

Sports and Work Injuries

What is the continuum of exertional heat illness?

Heat stress → heat cramps → heat exhaustion → heat stroke

What factors increase the risk for heat illness?

Vigorous activity, wet clothing, poor conditioning, obesity, medications that effect the autonomic nervous system, extremes of age, diuretic supplements, poor acclimatization

The symptoms of weakness, sweating, flushing, piloerection, headache, and dyspnea suggest what heat syndrome?

Heat exhaustion

The presence of central nervous system changes makes you concerned for what heat syndrome?

Heat stroke

A core temperature greater than what is diagnostic for heat stroke?

>104°F (>40°C)

What is the treatment for heat exhaustion?

Moderate cooling and oral hydration

What is the treatment for heat stroke?

Rapid cooling with ice packs and baths, intravenous (IV) fluids and urgent transport to medical facility

What is the initial treatment of frostbite to help prevent further tissue damage?

Rapid rewarming in hot bath at 40°C

What are absolute contraindications to exercise in pregnancy?

Preterm labor, ruptured membranes, incompetent cervix, poor fetal growth, pregnancy-induced hypertension, multiple gestation, persistent bleeding after 12 weeks

How do you calculate maximum heart rate (HR_{max}) for aerobic exercise?

$HR_{max}= 220 - age$

What is the calculation to determine target heart rate (THR)?

$THR = ([HR_{max} - resting\ heart\ rate] \times \% \ of\ desired\ training\ intensity) + resting\ heart\ rate$

What is the THR for increasing aerobic capacity?

70% of the maximum heart rate

HEAD INJURIES

Poor coordination, decreased attention span, emotional lability, retrograde amnesia, or anterograde amnesia can be signs of what head injury?

Concussion

Athletes with a concussion may complain of what symptoms after the initial injury?

Headache, dizziness, nausea, photophobia, phonophobia, decreased concentration, sleep disturbance, and impaired academic performance

The initial assessment of a sports head injury involves what steps on the field?

Check ABCs, palpate head and neck to rule out head or cervical spine injury

Once the on-field assessment is complete, what other assessment is needed in a head injury?

How injury occurred, estimation of force of impact, duration of symptoms, any previous concussions, neurological assessment, cognitive evaluation

Assessment of cognitive function at baseline and after a concussion resolves can be done with what testing?

Neuropsychological testing with measures of concentration, motor dexterity, information processing, visual and verbal memory, executive function, and brain stem function

What are the stages in activity for return to play?

Light aerobic exercise → moderate aerobic exercise → sport-specific drills → full contact activities → game play

What are the universally accepted guidelines about return to play after concussion?

There is no single guideline for making this decision, but they should not return until asymptomatic at rest or with any exertional maneuvers and should be on no medication that would minimize the signs or symptoms of concussion.

What assessment tool is indicated to help in the assessment of concussion, and includes symptom scale, mental status tests, instructions on neurologic screening, and guidelines for return to play?	Sport Concussion Assessment Tool (SCAT2)
What should you do with a contaminated tooth after avulsion during sports-related trauma in a conscious athlete?	Gently rinse then either reinsert, place in buccal sulcus or place in milk; immediate referral to dentist

SPRAINS AND STRAINS

What is the difference between a sprain and a strain?	Sprain: stretching of a ligament or joint capsule Strain: partial tear of muscle-tendon unit
What is the typical history reported by a patient with an acute sprain?	Sudden trauma or fall with "pop" or "snap" followed by pain, swelling, ecchymosis, or difficulty weight-bearing
What is the typical history in a patient with a muscle strain?	Sudden stretch on a muscle while it is actively contracting; if severe, can be associated with a "snapping" sensation
What is the treatment for an acute sprain?	**PRICEMMMS** **P**rotection **R**elative rest **I**ce **C**ompression **E**levation **M**edication **M**odalities Range of **M**otion **S**trength

What grade ankle sprains do the following descriptions describe?

Minimal swelling, little to no ecchymosis, minimal decreased range of motion (ROM)	Grade 1
Moderate "goose-egg" swelling, generalized tenderness, mild ecchymosis, and decreased ROM	Grade 2
Diffuse swelling, blurring of Achilles margin, medial ecchymosis, greatly decreased ROM	Grade 3

FRACTURES AND DISLOCATIONS

What symptoms are suggestive of a fracture in a patient?

Swelling, pain with movement, deformity, functional impairment, focal bony tenderness

If a person has a laceration of the skin over or near the fracture site, what type of fracture is it?

Open fracture

Name the fracture described by the following descriptions.

Fracture perpendicular to the shaft of bone

Transverse

Fracture line at an angle to the shaft

Oblique

A fracture with more than two fragments

Comminuted

Fracture line crosses the articular cartilage into the joint

Intra-articular

One cortex of the bone buckles without breaking, usually distal radius of ulna, often in kids

Torus

Fracture fragments are out of their usual alignment

Displaced

A gap exists between the proximal and distal segments of the fracture

Distracted

Angular deformity of a bone without a complete fracture

Greenstick

The day after a new femur fracture, a patient is found to be confused and short of breath. On examination, the patient is dyspneic and has a scattered pin-point rash. What is the most likely diagnosis?

Fat embolism syndrome

How are growth plate fractures in children classified?

Salter-Harris fractures. I: physis (growth plate), II: metaphysis and physis, III: epiphysis and physis, IV: all three, V: crush injury to physis

What Salter-Harris fractures require surgical repair to prevent future complications?

Types III, IV, and V

What are the risk factors for fracture nonunion?

Smoking, infection, malnutrition, NSAID overuse, poor immobilization, fracture location with poor blood supply

What are the four Rs for treatment of fractures?

Recognition
Reduction
Retention of reduction with a splint, cast, or fixation
Rehabilitation

What is the risk of casting a patient directly following an acute fracture?

Affected site can swell, making the cast too tight and risking a vascular or nerve injury or compartment syndrome

What are considerations in the radiographic evaluation of a long bone fracture?

Image joints above and below fracture site to look for dislocation, obtain images in at least two planes at 90° to each other (AP and lateral)

What additional images should you consider in children with an extremity fracture?

Views of asymptomatic limb, since open physes can make it difficult to identify fracture

What orthopedic injuries require immediate consultation?

Fracture with vascular injury and pelvic ring injuries

What injuries require orthopedic care within 6 hours of the initial injury?

Hip dislocation, open fracture, penetrating joint injury, compartment syndromes

What is the name for a bony projection without a secondary ossification center, where a muscle attaches?

Apophysis

What is the most commonly fractured long bone in children?

Clavicle

What is the major risk for an infant with a clavicle fracture at birth?

Brachial nerve palsy

What type of fracture is most typically associated with the following scenarios?

A child falls on an outstretched hand

Distal radius fracture, scaphoid fracture in older children and adolescents

A 3-year-old girl refused to bend her elbow after being lifted by her hand

Radial head subluxation (Nursemaid elbow)

A 24-year-old male punches a wall and fractures his right fifth metacarpal neck

Boxer fracture

A female raises her arms in self-defense, and her left arm absorbs the blow of a blunt object

Ulnar shaft fracture (Nightstick fracture)

Name the risks and/or complications associated with the following injuries:

Supracondylar fracture of the humerus

Volkmann ischemic contracture, brachial artery at risk

Mid-shaft humerus fracture

Risk of injury to radial nerve and resulting wrist drop and loss of thumb abduction

Proximal third scaphoid fracture in hand

Avascular necrosis (AVN)/nonunion due to disruption of blood supply

Boxer's fracture with skin laceration from punching someone in the jaw

Infection with oral pathogens, such as Eikenella. Treat with surgical irrigation, debridement, and IV antibiotics.

Nonpathologic fracture of proximal humerus

Frozen shoulder (early ROM exercises when pain improves, out of sling early)

Fifth metatarsal stress fracture

Nonunion of bone fragments

Tibial fracture

Acute compartment syndrome

LOWER LEG, FOOT, AND ANKLE INJURIES

What is the most common type of ankle sprain, characterized by pain anterior and inferior to the lateral malleolus?

Lateral sprain from an inversion injury, anterior talofibular ligament (ATFL) > posterior talofibular ligament (PTFL) > calcaneofibular

What additional injury do you need to worry about with a grade 3 ankle sprain?

Lateral malleolus fracture

Improper use of crutches can result in what injuries?

Axillary artery or venous thrombosis, radial nerve compression neuropathy

What are the guidelines for fitting crutches to a patient?

Length of crutch should be 75% of the patient's height, position crutch 4-6 in anterior and lateral to little toe, place handgrips even with the hips so arm is 30° flexed, tops of crutches should be 2 in below the armpits

What are the Ottawa ankle rules for when to order an ankle radiograph?

Order AP, PA, and mortise view x-ray, if pain is near the malleoli plus either inability to bear weight for immediately or in the emergency department (ED) for four steps, or tenderness at or within 6 cm above either malleolus

What are the Ottawa guidelines for when a radiograph is needed for a foot injury?

Pain in the mid-foot and either inability to bear weight for four steps or bone tenderness at navicular or base of fifth metatarsal

In what cases can you not use the Ottawa rules to guide your decision to obtain radiographs of an injured extremity?

Children below 18, pregnancy, multiple painful injuries, injury or intoxication that prevents examination

What is the most likely injury associated with the following scenarios?

Football player plants his foot just as another player hits his heel forcing further dorsiflexion, and he notices tenderness and swelling when moving his MTP joint

Turf toe (1st MTP sprain)

Middle-aged weekend warrior hears audible pop while jogging, absent plantar flexion in response to Thompson test (with the patient prone, squeeze the gastrocnemius), can't toe stand

Achilles tendon rupture

35-year-old male, training for marathon, with pain in proximal-medial aspect of calf, with swelling, ecchymosis, and tenderness, can't stand on toes

Gastrocnemius tear

Fracture to the proximal diaphysis near the base of the fifth metatarsal

Jones fracture

Pain with activity, abnormal stress with normal bone, commonly in individuals in sports and military recruits

Stress fracture: metatarsals (50%), calcaneous (25%), tibia (20%), tarsal navicular (<5%, especially in basketball players)

What is the name for postero-medial tibial pain, brought on by activity, and improved by rest?

Medial tibial stress syndrome (MTSS), often referred to as "shin splints"

What are the risk factors for the development of MTSS?

Pes planus (flat feet), rapid growth, hyperpronation

A 35-year-old female complains of pain on the surface of her heel and inside of her foot, which is worse after sitting or when she begins to walk in the morning. She does high-impact aerobics three times a week, and does not remember when she got her last pair of gym shoes. On examination, her pain increases with passive dorsiflexion. What is the most likely diagnosis?

Plantar Fasciitis

What is the etiology of the above diagnosis?

Inflammation of plantar aponeurosis

What are some common causes of the above diagnosis?

Increasing weekly mileage when running, use of inappropriate footwear, obesity

"Pain out of proportion" to the injury is characteristic of what injury?

Compartment syndromes

What are the other characteristic symptoms in the affected extremity?

Pain on passive motion of fingers or toes, pallor, paresthesias, pulselessness, paralysis of affected limb

What are the causes of acute compartment syndromes?

Fracture, crush injury, vascular injury, drug overdose, burn, trauma

What is the treatment for acute compartment syndrome?

Emergent fasciotomy

What groups of patients are often affected by chronic compartment syndromes?

Long-distance runners and new military recruits

What muscle compartment is most commonly affected by exertional compartment syndrome?

Anterior compartment of leg

What is the most common cause of medial ankle pain often associated with flat foot deformity?

Posterior tibial tendonitis

KNEE INJURIES

What are the indications for an x-ray series for a knee injury?

Any one of the following: point tenderness over patella, tenderness at head of fibula, inability to flex beyond 90°, inability to bear weight both immediately and at time of visit (4 steps), age >55

What are the key musculoskeletal differential diagnoses of acute knee pain?

Anterior cruciate ligament (ACL) tear, patellar dislocation, patellar fracture, lateral cruciate ligament (LCL)/ midclavicular line (MCL), posterior cruciate ligament (PCL), meniscal tear

What is the differential diagnosis of chronic anterior knee pain?

Patellofemoral dysfunction, Osgood-Schlatter disease, osteochondritis dessicans, patellar tendonitis, bursitis, patellar stress fracture

What direction is the patella most likely to dislocate?

Lateral >> medial

A 9-year-old boy presents with pain when squatting down to catch the baseball. He has been playing football 3 days a week and baseball twice a week. He is tender over the tibial tubercle. What is the likely diagnosis?

Osgood-Schlatter disease (OSD)

What is the treatment?

Decrease activity for 1-2 years (most children will grow out of it). Specialized neoprene bracing can provide symptomatic relief.

What is the knee injury most typical
for each history?

Popping sensation initially,   Meniscus tear (medial > lateral)
followed by sensation of locking
and lack of full extension

Female soccer player felt a pop in   ACL
her knee when she rotated on a
planted foot while running

A 17-year-old football player hit on   MCL
the lateral side of his leg by the
helmet of the tackling player,
causing valgus stress to knee joint.

A basketball player takes a hard,   PCL
direct fall onto her flexed knee. Or,
the driver of a car strikes his tibia
into the dashboard during a head-
on collision

Often referred to as the "unhappy   ACL, MCL, medial meniscus tears
triad" from being clipped from the
side in football, soccer, or other
contact sport

A 28-year-old runner presents to your   Iliotibial band (ITB) syndrome
office describing lateral knee pain,
especially when running downhill,
that goes away at rest. He can hear an
occasional pop when he is running. On
examination, he is tender to palpation
over the lateral femoral condyle, and
has pain when hopping with a flexed
knee. What is the likely diagnosis?

Name the physical examination test
used in the evaluation of ITB
syndrome described below.

With the patient lying down and   Noble compression test; pain at 30° is a
knee flexed to 90°, apply pressure to   positive test.
ITB over lateral femoral condyle
while extending the knee.

Patient lies on unaffected side with   Ober test; positive if leg remains
knee and hip flexed. Flex the   abducted indicating tight IT band
affected knee to 90° and abduct and
hyperextend hip while stabilizing
the pelvis. Lower the affected leg as
far as possible

| What is the treatment of ITB syndrome? | Physical therapy to improve hamstring and ITB flexibility, nonsteroid anti-inflammatory drugs (NSAIDs), ice, modifications to activity |

| What are some risk factors for ITB tightness? | Repetitive flexion and extension of the knee, long-distance running or cycling, genu varum, excessive foot pronation, internal tibial rotation |

Name the soft tissue injury most commonly associated with the following clinical scenarios?

| Painful swelling in calf and history of bump on back of knee | Ruptured Baker cyst (popliteal cyst) |

| Pain on repeated kneeling, with palpable area of swelling between patella and tibial tuberosity, often seen in tilers, roofers who work w/o kneepads | Prepatellar bursitis (Housemaid knee) |

| What is the name for diffuse knee pain associated with abnormal tracking of the patella through normal ROM, often seen in running, basketball, and soccer? | Patellofemoral dysfunction (PFD) |

| What is the treatment? | Rest, NSAIDs, correct the quadriceps imbalance by strengthening the vastus medialis oblique (VMO) |

| What traction apophysitis of the tibial tubercle is associated with trauma to an unclosed ossification system, and occurs in 9-15-year-old boys > girls? | Osgood-Schlatter disease |

BACK INJURIES

| In patients under the age of 50, what is the leading cause of disability? | Lower back pain |

| What is the differential diagnosis of lower back pain? | Refer to the table on next page: |

The Differential Diagnosis of Lower Back Pain

Diagnosis	Anatomy and Mechanism	Patient Description	Abnormal Tests
Back strain	Stretching or partial tearing of muscle or ligament fibers	Young to middle-aged patient with back ache and spasm, limited range of motion, local tenderness	None
Herniated disc	Gelatinous center of disc (nucleus pulposus) protrudes through the disc's fibrocartilaginous outer rim (annulus fibrosus) and through nerve root canal causing impingement	Middle-aged patient with sharp, shooting pain to buttock and leg, weakness and paresthesias, asymmetric reflexes	Herniation seen on MRI, localized by myelography
Spondylolisthesis	Anterior displacement of vertebra	Presents at any age with lordosis; stiff back; pain in lower back, thighs, and buttocks; tight hamstrings	XRs show possible fracture
Spinal stenosis	Narrowing of spinal canal and nerve root canals, intervertebral foramina secondary to spondylosis	>50 years, "pins and needles" sensation and shooting pain increased by walking up an incline and decreased by sitting	XRs may show findings consistent with OA/ spondylosis
Ankylosing spondylitis	Chronic inflammation of intervertebral and sacroiliac joints, vertebrae may fuse	Young adult male with tenderness of SI joints and decreased back flexion	XRs show sacroiliac (SI) joint narrowing and sclerosis, fusion of vertebral bodies appears as "bamboo spine"

With the exception of ankylosing spondylitis, what is the treatment for acute lower back pain without neurologic, systemic symptoms, or radicular findings?

Conservative management: NSAIDs, stretching and strengthening, relative rest, and physical therapy. Surgery is rarely needed.

What is the differential diagnosis of lower back pain in children and adolescents?

Muscle strain, spondylolysis, sacroiliac dysfunction, scoliosis, malignancy, infection (osteomyelitis, paraspinal abscess), vertebral fracture, ankylosing spondylitis, Reiter syndrome

What is the name for lower back pain caused by an abnormally increased kyphosis of the thoracolumbar spine that doesn't correct with hyperextension and is seen in adolescents?

Scheuermann disease

What is the radiographic finding associated with this diagnosis?

Greater than 5° of anterior wedging of at least three adjacent vertebral bodies

What is the treatment for mild disease?

Bracing and physical therapy

What is the treatment for severe disease?

Spinal fusion

What is the preferred imaging modality to evaluate scoliosis?

PA radiographs

Is screening indicated for scoliosis in adolescents?

No

When is MRI indicated for the evaluation of scoliosis in kids?

Onset prior to 8 years old, rapid curve progression greater than 1° per month, left thoracic curve, neurologic deficit, or pain

What is the location of the fracture seen in spondylolysis?

Pars interarticularis

What is the classic exam finding in spondylolysis?

Pain with extension of the back with single leg loading in the presence of normal neurologic exam

What are the risk factors for malignancy associated with lower back pain?

Personal history of cancer, age >50 years, pain not relieved by rest, pain that worsens at night or wakes patient from sleep, symptoms longer than 4 weeks, constitutional symptoms

In the absence of risk factors for malignancy or neurologic findings, when is imaging indicated for lower back pain?

Failure of conservative treatment for 2-4 weeks

HIP AND GROIN INJURIES

Name the soft tissue injury most commonly associated with the following clinical scenario?

Pain in hip after a direct blow that increases with rotation or with lateral bending

Iliac crest bone contusion (hip pointer)

Runner started running stairs to prepare for upcoming climbing trip. Point tenderness posterior to greater trochanter, pain with resisted abduction, and lateral thigh rotation

Trochanteric bursitis

What is the most common site for a thigh hematoma?

Quadriceps

An osteoporotic woman slips, hears a snap, and is unable to bear weight. She reports it is very painful. On examination, you don't notice any swelling, but see that her left lower limb is externally rotated and noticeably shorter than the right. What are you worried about?

Avascular necrosis (AVN) and deep vein thrombosis (DVT) with a femoral neck fracture

In addition to management of her fracture, what additional medical therapy would you recommend?

Anticoagulate to decrease risk of DVT while in the hospital, bone health evaluation, appropriate medication prior to discharge (calcium, vitamin D, bisphosphonate)

What is the most common cause of a limp in toddlers?

Infected joint (septic joint, osteomyelitis, toxic synovitis)

What is the initial workup for a child that presents with a limp?

Radiographs of affected joint and above and below joint, complete blood count (CBC), erythrocyte sedimentation rate (ESR), C-reactive protein (CRP)

What are the most common causes of a limp in adolescents and teens?

Slipped capital femoral epiphysis (SCFE), juvenile rheumatoid arthritis (JRA), avascular necrosis of the femoral head (Legg-Calve-Perthes disease)

A mother brings in her 6-year-old son who presents with 2 months of a painless limp, along with complaints of mild knee pain. On examination, you notice that he has limited internal rotation, and the affected leg appears smaller than the other. What diagnosis do you suspect?

Legg-Calve-Perthes disease

What is the etiology of this disease?

Avascular necrosis of the femoral head of unknown etiology

What is the treatment of this disease?

Observation, if mild; bracing or hip abduction with a Petrie cast, if moderate; osteotomy, if severe

What occurs when acute or repetitive microtraumas cause the femoral head to shear off the femoral neck prior to epiphyseal closure, and causes painful abduction and lateral rotation?

SCFE (slipped capital femoral epiphysis)

What are the risk factors for this condition?

Obesity, male gender, African American ethnicity, history of hypothyroidism, 10-14 years old

What radiographic views should you order when you suspect this diagnosis?

Radiographs of both hips in AP and frog-leg lateral to look for posterior and medial displacement of the femoral head

What is the underlying dysfunction associated with a snapping hip from repetitive hip flexion?

Iliopsoas dysfunction or tendinitis

Pain in the groin or buttock associated with popping clicking and catching suggests what injury?

Acetabular labral tear

Acute posterior proximal leg/gluteal pain after forcible flexion of the hip with the knee extended is characteristic of what injury?

Avulsion fracture of ischial tuberosity at proximal attachment of biceps femoris and semitendinosus (Hurdler injury)

In what activities is this injury most likely to occur?

Acceleration sports such as sprinting, soccer, basketball, and martial arts

SHOULDER INJURIES

What is the injury associated with the following scenarios?

Football player presents with a high-riding clavicle, tenderness at acromioclavicular (AC) joint and intact motor and sensory examinations	AC separation
An older patient describes poorly localized pain with activities, such as overhead lifting or throwing a baseball that has slowly worsened over the last year	Impingement syndrome, often secondary to rotator cuff tendinitis
A weight lifter is repeatedly bench pressing, and complains of pain and clicking when his arm goes through a full range of motion	Glenoid labral injury

What are the muscles of the rotator cuff?

SITS
Supraspinatus
Infraspinatus
Teres minor
Subscapularis

What are four indications of a probable rotator cuff tear?

1. Supraspinatus weakness
2. Weak external rotation
3. Positive impingement sign
4. Advanced age

What are the bony attachments of the rotator cuff muscles?

They all attach the scapula to the lateral humeral head.

What imaging modality can best identify a rotator cuff injury?

Magnetic resonance imaging (MRI)

What imaging findings will you see in a rotator cuff injury?

Swollen tendon or tear in rotator cuff, with rare calcium deposits on radiographs if chronic rotator cuff tendonitis

What is the treatment for a patient with suspected rotator cuff tendonitis?

NSAIDs and refraining from overhead activities, with a subacromial corticosteroid injection, if symptoms persist

What is the treatment of a mild, proximal clavicular fracture?

Sling to immobilize for 3-4 weeks

What fracture is associated with an anterior glenohumeral dislocation?

Posterolateral humeral head fracture

What is the most common type of shoulder dislocation, usually from a fall on an outstretched arm?

Anterior shoulder dislocation

How will a patient with this type of dislocation typically present?

Affected arm abducted and externally rotated

What type of shoulder dislocation is associated with seizures and electrocutions?

Posterior shoulder dislocation

ELBOW, HAND, AND WRIST INJURIES

Name the soft tissue injury most commonly associated with the following clinical scenarios?

Elbow pain reproduced by resisted wrist or middle finger extension

Lateral epicondylitis (tennis elbow)

Elbow pain from overuse of flexor pronator, made worse by wrist flexion

Medial epicondylitis (golfer's elbow or little league elbow)

Acute onset of medial elbow pain after throwing, worst at acceleration phase

Ulnar collateral ligament sprain

Posterior elbow pain at terminal extension while throwing

Posterior impingement

What is the most common carpal fracture in the hand?

Scaphoid fracture

How is the diagnosis of a scaphoid fracture made?

Fracture on radiographs, or clinical suspicion and tenderness in the anatomical snuff box. Radiographs may take 10-14 days to reveal the fracture.

What is the treatment of an uncomplicated scaphoid fracture?

Thumb spica cast for 12 weeks

With a distal interphalangeal (DIP) joint fracture, when do you need to use open reduction/internal fixation (ORIF) to avoid degenerative change?

If >30% of the articular surface is involved

Name the injury most commonly associated with the following clinical scenarios?

A teenage softball player hurt her finger while catching a ball yesterday. On examination, she is tender over the distal interphalangeal (DIP), and unable to extend the joint fully, without evidence of fracture.	Ruptured distal extensor tendon at distal phalanx (mallet finger)
What is the treatment?	Splint DIP joint continuously for 6 weeks
A football player hyperextends his fourth right finger while tackling an opposing player during practice today, and now has bruising and tenderness over the entire volar aspect of his finger and cannot flex the DIP.	Avulsion of flexor digitorum profundus (jersey finger)
What is the treatment?	Splint finger and immediate orthopedic referral
A patient presents 2 weeks after a forced flexion injury of the proximal interphalangeal (PIP) joint. He did not see a doctor initially, but now presents with a flexion deformity of his PIP joint.	Central slip tear of the extensor mechanism proximal to PIP (Boutonniere deformity)
What is the treatment?	Splint PIP in full extension for 6 weeks
What is the treatment of a mild collateral ligament sprain of the PIP joint, with no fracture on x-ray, and slight laxity?	Buddy taping to adjacent finger for 6 weeks, NSAIDs for symptomatic relief
A patient presents to your office with swelling at the base of her thumb, and pain that is worse when she tries to make a fist or move her thumb. She has lost strength in her grip and ROM in her thumb. What is the most likely diagnosis?	De Quervain tenosynovitis
What tendons are involved in this condition?	Abductor pollicis longus, extensor brevis
What physical examination test is diagnostic?	Finkelstein test: full flexion of thumb in the palm, then ulnar deviation of the wrist
What group of patients is most commonly affected?	Middle-aged women
What is the treatment?	Thumb spica splint and 2-week course of NSAIDs, with corticosteroid injection if no improvement

What nerve is entrapped at the wrist in carpal tunnel syndrome (CTS)?	Median nerve
What conditions can precipitate CTS?	Overuse trauma, diabetes mellitus, thyroid dysfunction, pregnancy, rheumatoid arthritis
What is the differential diagnosis of pain and paresthesias in the wrist?	Arthritis, cervical radiculopathy at C6, ulnar neuropathy, ganglion cyst, hypothyroidism, diabetic neuropathy, flexor carpi radialis tenosynovitis
What group of people does carpal tunnel most often affect?	Middle-aged or pregnant women
Where do patients typically report paresthesias or numbness?	Median nerve distribution: palmar aspect of thumb, index finger, long finger, and half of the ring finger
What daily tasks will patients with carpal tunnel often complain of trouble with?	Opening jars, grasping objects, twisting lids, driving, reading
Aside from the wrist, where do patients often report aching in CTS?	Proximal forearm and in some cases the shoulder
What physical examination findings can suggest a diagnosis of CTS?	Thenar atrophy, weakness of thenar muscles, positive provocative test
Identify the name of the following clinical tests used in the diagnosis of CTS?	
Have the patients place the wrists in flexion and look for aching or numbness in the median nerve distribution within 60 seconds	Phalen maneuver
The examiner uses his thumb to put pressure over the median nerve at the wrist for up to 30 seconds, looking for either pain or numbness in the median nerve distribution	Durken carpal compression test
The examiner taps over the median nerve at the wrist and looks for tingling in some or all digits in the median nerve distribution	Tinel sign
How is the diagnosis of CTS made?	Clinical history and physical examination; electrophysiologic testing only to confirm, if needed

What is the treatment of mild cases of CTS?

Splinting in neutral position at night and as tolerated during the day, NSAIDs, ergonomic modifications to keyboards if work-related

If conservative treatment fails, what other therapies can be considered?

Corticosteroid injection to carpal canal

What are the indications for referral in CTS?

Failed nonsurgical treatment for 3 months or persistent sensory loss

What is the treatment of CTS in pregnancy?

Splinting or corticosteroid injection (since most cases resolve after delivery)

CHAPTER 19

Breast Masses, Breast Pain, and Nipple Discharge

BREAST MASS

On breast exam, which positions are used to aid with the inspection of breasts?

Seated with arms to the side, arms over the head (to expose the lateral and inferior aspects of the breast), hands pressed against hips (contracting the pectoral muscles can cause dimpling of the skin suggesting that a tumor has entrapped a Cooper ligament)

What can be observed while visually inspecting breasts?

Symmetry; breast contour looking for masses, skin retraction, or skin dimpling; skin color and texture

During the breast exam, when should lymph nodes be palpated?

When the patient is seated, the axillary fat pad moves anterior exposing the axillary lymph nodes (but don't forget to palpate the infraclavicular and supraclavicular lymph nodes as well).

Describe the examination of breasts while the patient is supine.

The patient's ipsilateral arm should be placed above the head. Palpate the breast tissue with the second, third, and fourth finger pads. Other hand supports the breast tissue. Move finger pads in a systematic fashion (spiral pattern from the nipple to the outer breast or a vertical strip pattern). Compress each nipple between your thumb and index fingers, and inspect for discharge. Examine the contralateral side.

In which quadrant is breast cancer typically found?	Upper, outer quadrant
What two entities comprise breast lumps?	1. Cysts 2. Solid masses
What are the questions to ask when evaluating a patient with a breast lump?	Personal history of breast cancer, prior breast biopsy (especially one indicating atypical hyperplasia), risk factors for breast cancer (age, family history of breast cancer, age of menarche, age at first pregnancy, age at menopause, alcohol use, hormone replacement therapy), relationship with menstrual cycle, breast pain, nipple discharge
What percentage of women born in the United States will develop breast cancer at some time in their lives?	12.7% (1 in 8)
According to the National Cancer Institute's Surveillance, Epidemiology, and End Results Program, what are the odds of developing breast cancer for 30-39 year olds?	1 in 233
What are the odds of developing breast cancer for 60-69 year olds?	1 in 27
What percentage of all breast cancers is associated with inherited genetic mutations?	5%-6% (most of the mutations involve BRCA1 and BRCA2)
According to the US Preventive Services Task Force, who should be offered testing for BRCA mutations?	
For non-Ashkenazi Jewish women	Anybody with two 1st-degree relatives with breast cancer (at least one diagnosed at age ≤50); a combination of three or more 1st- or 2nd-degree relatives with breast cancer, regardless of age at diagnosis; a combination of both breast and ovarian cancer among 1st- and 2nd-degree relatives; a 1st-degree relative with bilateral breast cancer; a combination of two or more 1st- or 2nd-degree relatives with ovarian cancer, regardless of age at diagnosis; a 1st- or 2nd-degree relative with both breast and ovarian cancer at any age; or history of breast cancer in a male relative
For women of Ashkenazi Jewish descent	Any 1st-degree relative (or two 2nd-degree relatives on the same side of the family) with breast or ovarian cancer

What are the options for breast and ovarian cancer surveillance and/or prophylaxis in patients with BRCA1 or BRCA2 mutations?

There are three options (though many areas of controversy exist): increased surveillance (mammography, breast MRI, clinical/self-breast exams, transvaginal ultrasounds, and serum CA-125 levels), chemoprevention (tamoxifen and oral contraception pills), riskreducing surgery (bilateral mastectomy and bilateral salpingooporectomy)

What is the role of ultrasound in evaluating breast lumps?

It distinguishes cysts from masses and determines whether a mammographically suspicious mass is amenable to ultrasound-guided biopsy.

What are the types of breast cysts?

Simple cysts (benign), complicated cysts (rarely malignant [0.4%]), complex cysts (contain cystic and solid components, 20%-43% represent cancer)

What are other benign causes of breast lumps?

Fibroadenomas, ductal hyperplasia without atypia, papilloma (can contain areas of atypia or ductal carcinoma in situ), sclerosis adenosis, atypical hyperplasia (associated with increased risk of breast cancer)

What are fibroadenomas?

Firm, painless, mobile masses that increase in size during pregnancy or with estrogen and regress after menopause

What are the ways of obtaining biopsies of palpable or nonpalpable breast lesions?

Fine needle aspiration (for cystic lesions), fine needle aspiration biopsy (for solid masses), core needle biopsy (larger gauge needle compared to fine needle aspiration), excisional biopsy, incisional biopsy (if the mass is too large to excise)

What is the role of mammogram in evaluating a palpable breast lump?

Identifies other suspicious areas in either breast that might affect management

What is the most common type of breast cancer?

Infiltrating ductal cancer (80%)

What are other types of breast cancer?

Infiltrating lobular, Paget disease, inflammatory carcinoma

For which type of breast cancer is the overlying skin described as *peau d' orange* (orange peel)?	Inflammatory carcinoma
Which type of breast cancer is associated with nipple eczema and bloody nipple discharge?	Paget disease
What is the difference between in situ and infiltrating carcinoma?	The tumor cells of in situ carcinomas remain within the ducts or lobules and do not invade the surrounding stroma.
What percentage of breast masses are mammographically occult?	20% (suspicious masses should still be biopsied even after negative mammograms)
Why are mammograms less useful in women under 35 years of age?	Their breast tissue is frequently too dense to adequately evaluate lumps

BREAST PAIN

What percentage of women with breast cancer present with breast pain?	1.2%-6.7%
What are the features of cyclical breast pain?	Pain is worse during the week prior to the onset of menses, pain resolves with the onset of menses, bilateral pain, pain is worse in the upper outer quadrant
What hormones have been associated with cyclical breast pain?	Estrogen and prolactin (which stimulate ductal elements), progesterone (which stimulates breast stroma)
Cyclical breast pain is comprised of which conditions?	Cyclical mastalgia, nodular sensitive breasts (formerly fibrocystic breast disease, but because the changes are a normal response to hormones, the term "disease" can be misleading)
What are features of noncyclical breast pain?	Unilateral; variable location of pain; not associated with menstrual cycles

What are causes of noncyclical breast pain?

Ductal ectasia, mastitis (most common in lactating women during the first month postpartum), inflammatory breast cancer, hidradenitis suppurativa, pregnancy, thrombophlebitis, prior breast surgery, medications (eg, hormone replacement therapy), trauma

What imaging modalities can assist with determining the cause of breast pain?

Ultrasound, mammogram

What are supportive treatments for breast pain?

Well-fitting bra, warm compresses, low fat/high complex carbohydrate diet, oral and topical NSAIDs, danazol, tamoxifen. Caffeine avoidance, evening primrose oil, and vitamin supplementation appear to be ineffective.

NIPPLE DISCHARGE

What are the types of nipple discharge?

Milk, physiologic nipple discharge (galactorrhea), pathologic nipple discharge

What are the typical characteristics of galactorrhea?

Bilateral, white or clear discharge (though unilateral galactorrhea is also possible)

What are the most common causes of galactorrhea?

Hyperprolactinemia from a pituitary adenoma or medications such as atypical antipsychotics

What characteristics suggest that the nipple discharge is from a pathologic etiology?

Unilateral, persistent, spontaneous, and frequently sanguinous discharge

What is the most common cause of pathologic nipple discharge?

Papilloma

What are other causes of pathologic nipple discharge?

Ductal ectasia, fibrocystic breast changes, breast cancer

Which patients with nipple discharge should be evaluated by a surgeon?

Patients with a palpable breast mass, abnormal breast imaging, guaiac positive or grossly bloody discharge, or spontaneous/uniductal discharge

CHAPTER 20

Abdominal Pain

What is the differential diagnosis of pain in the following locations?

Right upper quadrant (RUQ)

Biliary disease, colitis, hepatic abscess or mass, pulmonary infection or embolus, renal stone or infection, pelvic inflammatory disease with liver capsule inflammation (Fitz-Hugh-Curtis syndrome)

Epigastric

Myocardial infarction (MI) or pericarditis, biliary disease, esophagitis, gastritis or peptic ulcer, pancreatic mass or pancreatitis, aortic dissection, mesenteric ischemia

Right lower quadrant (RLQ)

Appendicitis, colitis, irritable bowel syndrome/inflammatory bowel disease (IBS/IBD) or diverticulitis, ectopic pregnancy, fibroids, ovarian mass, ovarian torsion, pelvic inflammatory disease (PID), nephrolithiasis or pyelonephritis, hernia

Left lower quadrant (LLQ)

Diverticulitis, colitis, or sigmoid volvulus; ectopic pregnancy, fibroids, ovarian mass, ovarian torsion, PID; nephrolithiasis or pyelonephritis; hernia

Abdominal wall

Muscle strain, herpes zoster, hernia

What are unusual causes for acute abdominal pain in a patient without obvious cause?

Narcotic withdrawal, sickle cell crisis, porphyria, heavy metal poisoning

What are the risk factors for pancreatic cancer?

Smoking, family history of pancreatic cancer, history of pancreatitis, diabetes mellitus

What are the typical presenting symptoms of pancreatic cancer?

Painless jaundice, depression, weight loss, abdominal pain later in disease

What are the most common risk factors for pancreatitis in the United States?	Alcohol use and gallstones
A normal white blood cell count rules out appendicitis. True or false?	False
What is the imaging study of choice for evaluating patients with acute right upper quadrant abdominal pain?	Ultrasonography
What is the imaging study of choice for evaluating patients with acute right lower quadrant or left lower quadrant abdominal pain?	Computed tomography
What is the imaging test of choice for evaluating pregnant women with right lower quadrant pain?	Ultrasonography
In what circumstances are plain radiographs of the abdomen helpful in the evaluation of abdominal pain?	Detecting free air under diaphragm, finding abnormal calcifications (such as kidney stones), diagnosing bowel obstruction with multiple dilated loops and air-fluid levels
What two tests combined are 95% sensitive for ectopic pregnancy?	1. Transvaginal ultrasonography 2. Human chorionic gonadotropin level greater than 25 mIU per mL
What is the classic finding in appendicitis?	RLQ pain, or migration of pain from the periumbilical area to the RLQ
What physical exam maneuvers are used to assess a patient with possible appendicitis?	Rovsing sign, Psoas sign, Obturator sign, pain at McBurney point (1/3 of the distance from the anterior superior iliac spine to the umbilicus)
What finding has the highest positive predictive value for a bowel obstruction?	Constipation
What is the name for sharp, localized abdominal pain that increases, peaks, and subsides and is associated with diseases of hollow viscera?	Colic

When a supine patient has increased pain upon lifting their head and shoulders off the exam table, what sign is positive?	Carnett sign
What are the classic findings in cholecystitis?	Murphy sign, RUQ pain, fever, and jaundice
What is the definition of constipation?	Passage of fewer than three stools in a week, often with passage of hard difficult to pass stools
What is the first-line treatment of constipation?	Increase intake of fluid, bulk food (cereal, vegetables), and pitted fruits and juices
What diagnosis do you not want to miss in a newborn with delayed passage of meconium or a child with chronic constipation?	Hirschsprung disease
What is intussusception?	Telescoping of one part of small bowel over another
What are the signs and symptoms?	Crampy abdominal pain, vomiting, blood and mucus in the stool (currant jelly stool)
What is the name for a true outpouching of the small bowel that has the potential to become inflamed, ulcerate/perforate, or cause bowel obstruction in children?	Meckel diverticulum
This finding is an embryologic remnant of what structure?	Omphalomesenteric duct
What is the "rule of twos" with regard to this diagnosis?	It occurs in 2% of population, is usually 2 in long, is located within 2 ft of the ileocecal valve, contains two types of tissue (gastric and pancreatic), and causes symptoms around 2 years of age.

GASTROESOPHAGEAL REFLUX DISEASE

What is gastroesophageal reflux disease (GERD)?	Pathologic reflux of acidic contents from the stomach into the esophagus causing symptoms or complications

What is physiologic reflux?

Reflux occurring after eating, for only short periods of time, and causing no symptoms

What is reflux esophagitis?

GERD along with esophageal inflammation on endoscopy or biopsy

What pathophysiologic factors may contribute to GERD?

Decreased resting tone of the lower esophageal sphincter, impaired clearance of acid from the esophagus, decreased mucosal protective mechanisms

What symptoms do patients with GERD typically complain of?

Heartburn, regurgitation of acidic material, dysphagia

When do symptoms of GERD typically occur?

After meals and when lying supine

What are some atypical symptoms of GERD?

Chest pain, water brash (hypersalivation), odynophagia, nausea, asthma, laryngitis, cough

What is the differential diagnosis of GERD?

Esophageal motility disorders, infectious esophagitis, pill esophagitis, coronary artery disease, gastritis, peptic ulcer disease, nonulcer dyspepsia, biliary tract disease

How are most cases of GERD diagnosed?

Clinical history and a therapeutic response to an antireflux regimen of lifestyle and dietary modifications and/or acid suppression medication

When should you consider including endoscopy in your diagnostic workup?

Odynophagia, bysphagia, weight loss, early satiety, bleeding, symptoms refractory to treatment

Who is a candidate for a 24-hour ambulatory esophageal pH monitoring?

No response to empiric medication and no evidence of inflammation on endoscopy

What are the complications of GERD?

Esophagitis, esophageal ulcers, strictures, Barrett esophagus, iron-deficiency anemia, extraesophageal manifestations such as asthma, cough, and laryngitis

What is Barrett esophagus?

Metaplasia from squamous to columnar epithelium in the lower esophagus resulting from chronic reflux

When should endoscopic surveillance for Barrett esophagus be considered?

Symptoms for longer than 5 years

Barrett esophagus puts patients at increased risk for what malignancy?

Adenocarcinoma of the esophagus in 10% of patients

Name the available treatment/ management for GERD under the following categories. (Note: remember that the therapy must be titrated to the severity of the symptoms.)

   Dietary modifications

Avoid large meals; avoid eating for 2-3 hours prior to reclining; avoid chocolate, cola, alcohol, coffee, and fatty food intake

   Lifestyle modifications

Elevate the head of the bed, weight loss (if obese), smoking cessation

   Avoidance of medications that may contribute to reflux

Oral bisphosphonates, calcium-channel blockers, anticholinergics, sedatives, theophylline

   Drug therapy to reduce acid

Antacids, H2-blockers, proton pump inhibitors (PPI)

What are the indications for antireflux surgery (Nissen fundoplication, etc)?

Persistent or recurrent symptoms refractory to medical management, severe esophagitis, Barrett esophagus, stricture, recurrent aspiration or pneumonia associated with GERD

PEPTIC ULCER DISEASE

What are the two major etiologies of peptic ulcer disease (PUD)?

1. *Helicobacter pylori (H. pylori)* infection
2. Nonsteroidal anti-inflammatory drug (NSAID) use

What symptoms do patients with PUD have?

Epigastric pain of a burning or gnawing quality that may radiate to the back

Pain that is relieved by food intake or antacids, but recurs 2-3 hours after meals and during the night on an empty stomach is classic for what diagnosis?

Duodenal ulcer

Pain that occurs very soon after meals and is less responsive to antacids is classic for what diagnosis?

Gastric ulcer

What are the complications of peptic ulcers?

Perforation, penetration, hemorrhage, pyloric outlet obstruction

What is the differential diagnosis of PUD?

Nonulcer dyspepsia (functional dyspepsia), drug-induced dyspepsia, gastric carcinoma, duodenal neoplasia, Crohn disease, granulomatous disease, gastric infections, duodenal infections

How is PUD diagnosed?

The clinical history raises suspicion for PUD, and confirmation can be made by upper endoscopy or a radiographic upper gastrointestinal (GI) series.

How is a peptic ulcer diagnosed by upper GI series?

Barium in a round or oval ulcer crater

If an upper GI series shows an ulcer within a mass protruding into the gastric lumen, an irregular filling defect in the ulcer crater and irregularity of the mucosal folds, what should you be concerned about?

Gastric cancer

H. pylori infection increases the risk of what malignancies?

Gastric adenocarcinoma and mucosa-associated lymphoid tissue (MALT) lymphoma, which frequently regresses with H. pylori eradication

What noninvasive tests are available to test patients for H. pylori infection?

Serum H. pylori IgG antibody serology (stays positive even after treatment), carbon-labeled urea breath testing, stool antigen testing

How is H. pylori infection eradicated?

PPI for acid suppression and antibiotics twice daily for 10-14 days (clarithromycin and amoxicillin or metronidazole)

When should PUD be managed surgically?

Peptic ulcers refractory to medical therapy; recurrent peptic ulcers; ulcer disease that is complicated by hemorrhage, penetration, perforation, or obstruction; duodenal ulcers greater than 5 cm in size

What is the basic goal of peptic ulcer surgery?	Selective vagotomy to denervate the acid-secreting parietal cells of the stomach
What is Zollinger-Ellison syndrome?	Hypersecretion of gastric acid caused by a gastrin-secreting islet cell tumor of the pancreas, resulting in multiple peptic ulcers that may be in unusual locations and are refractory to standard medical treatment or recurrent after surgery

GALLBLADDER DISEASE

Calcium gallstones are the most common type. True or false?	False. 80% are cholesterol stones
What are the risk factors for gallstones?	Age >40 years, female gender, pregnancy, oral contraceptive or estrogen replacement therapy, obesity, rapid weight loss, Native American ethnicity, family history of 1st degree relatives with gallstones, "Fat, female, forty, and fertile"
What is biliary colic?	Recurrent RUQ pain from the gallbladder contracting against a gallstone in the gallbladder outlet
Where does the pain from biliary colic radiate?	To the back or right shoulder
Can gallstones be seen on plain abdominal x-ray?	Only 10% of gallstones have enough calcium to be radiopaque
In patients with a typical history of biliary colic but no evidence of gallstones on ultrasound, what other diagnostic tools can be used?	CT of the abdomen, HIDA scan, bile microscopy, endoscopic ultrasound
How should patients with biliary colic and gallstones on ultrasound be treated?	Pain control with meperidine or NSAIDs, elective cholecystectomy
Why is meperidine preferred over morphine in patients with biliary symptoms?	It causes theoretical decreased Sphincter of Oddi spasm.

Is surgery indicated for the asymptomatic patient with incidental gallstones on ultrasound?	No
What is the implication of finding a calcified gallbladder (porcelain gallbladder) on imaging?	Increased risk of malignancy
What are the complications of gallstones?	Acute cholecystitis, ascending cholangitis, acute biliary pancreatitis, gallstone ileus, gallbladder cancer
What sign is positive when a patient has severe pain and inspiratory arrest with palpation in the area of the gallbladder?	Murphy sign
What are the key lab findings of acute cholecystitis?	Leukocytosis with a left shift
What ultrasound findings support a diagnosis of acute cholecystitis?	The presence of gallstones with gallbladder wall thickening, pericholecystic fluid, or a sonographic Murphy sign
How should acute cholecystitis be treated?	IV fluids, NPO status, pain control with opioids or ketorolac, empiric antibiotics, cholecystectomy
What is the name for cholecystitis in the absence of gallstones (5%-10%, or cases of acute cholecystitis)?	Acalculous cholecystitis
What groups of patients are especially at risk for this?	Critically ill patients or following major surgery or trauma, patients on total parenteral nutrition (TPN)
What is the name for the triad of fever, jaundice, and RUQ pain found in ascending cholangitis?	Charcot triad
What lab findings are consistent with ascending cholangitis?	Leukocytosis with left shift; elevated alkaline phosphatase, gammaglutamyl transpeptidase (GGT), and conjugated bilirubin
Reynold pentad of altered mental status, hypotension, fever, jaundice, and RUQ pain is found in what condition?	Supparative cholangitis

What percentage of patients with gallstone disease develop pancreatitis?   5%

What percentage of acute pancreatitis is caused by gallstones?   33%

In what patient population is gallstone ileus most common?   Elderly patients

CHAPTER 21

Diarrhea

What is encopresis?	Fecal soiling—often occurs with constipation as looser stool moves around an impaction
What is the most common infectious cause of diarrhea in infants?	Rotavirus
What is the mechanism of transmission?	Fecal-oral
In what season is this most common?	Winter
What are the symptoms associated with this infection?	Watery diarrhea, fever, vomiting, perhaps abdominal pain
What vaccines are recommended to prevent this infection?	RV5 (Rotateq) orally in a three-dose series at 2, 4, and 6 months of age or RV1 (Rotarix) orally in a two-dose series at 2 and 4 months of age
What are contraindications to the administration of vaccine?	History of severe allergic reaction to rotavirus vaccine; immunocompromised infants; infants with acute, moderate-to-severe gastrointestinal illness at the time of vaccination
Do the new approved vaccines cause intussusception?	Ongoing safety reports indicate there may be a risk of 0-4 cases in 100,000 people within the first 30 days of the vaccine, with most happening within the first week. However, the vaccine is still recommended while monitoring is ongoing.
What complication do you want to rule out when seeing a patient with diarrhea?	Dehydration

What are the signs of dehydration in an infant?

Elevated heart rate, lethargy, poor capillary refill, skin tenting, decreased urination, dry mucus membranes (eyes, oral mucosa)

What is the treatment for mild-to-moderate dehydration secondary to diarrhea?

Oral rehydration therapy (ORT); avoid sports drinks, sodas, and other sugary items

How do you usually administer ORT?

50-100 mL/kg over 4 hours initially, then 10 mL/kg for each additional stool

What are some signs of severe dehydration?

Rapid/weak pulses, decreased blood pressure, no urine output, very sunken eyes/fontanelles, dry mucus membranes, tented or mottled skin, delayed capillary refill

When are intravenous (IV) fluids required to treat dehydration secondary to diarrhea?

Severe dehydration, uncontrollable vomiting, inability to drink because of extreme fatigue or decreased level of consciousness, GI distention

What are some noninfectious causes of diarrhea in children?

Overfeeding, malabsorption, necrotizing enterocolitis (NEC), strangulated hernia, ovarian/testicular torsion, mesenteric thrombus

What factors in a patient's history suggest that diarrhea is infectious in etiology?

Ingestion of raw food, seafood, or picnic food; recent travel (foreign or camping); hospitalization, nursing home care, or day care; anal intercourse; IV drug use; sick contacts

What time course of a patient's diarrhea usually reflects an infectious etiology?

Acute diarrhea, with duration less than 2 weeks

What are the major bacterial causes of diarrhea?

Salmonella, Shigella, Staphylococcus aureus, Campylobacter, Escherichia coli, Yersinia enterocolitica, Vibrio parahaemolyticus, Vibrio cholerae, Bacillus cereus, Clostridium difficile

What are the major viral causes of diarrhea?

Rotavirus and caliciviruses (such as Norwalk virus)

What are the major parasitic causes of diarrhea?

Giardia, Entamoeba histolytica, Cryptosporidium

What is the usual etiologic agent of "traveler's diarrhea"?

Bacteria such as enterotoxigenic *E. coli*

How can travelers reduce their risk of developing diarrhea?

Avoid tap water, fruits, salads, uncooked or under-cooked foods, and other foods that may be contaminated; use of antibiotic prophylaxis is controversial

What is dysentery?

Bloody diarrhea containing mucus and polymorphonuclear leukocytes (inflammation of the colonic or ileal mucosa by invasion of organisms or toxin-induced injury)

What organisms cause dysentery?

Campylobacter, Salmonella, Shigella, E. coli O157:H7

Most cases of acute diarrhea are infectious and self-limited in nature. True or false?

True

How is acute diarrhea treated?

Patients without signs of systemic toxicity may be treated symptomatically (antidiarrheals, such as loperamide or bismuth subsalicylate) and with oral fluid and electrolyte replacement

What is the BRAT diet?

It is used to transition from liquid to solid diet after diarrhea; bananas, rice, applesauce, and toast.

How should you manage patients with bloody diarrhea, high fever, or signs of systemic toxicity?

Avoid antimotility agents, order stool studies (fecal leukocytes, bacterial culture, *C. difficile* toxin, and ova and parasites), start antibiotics

What is hemolytic uremic syndrome (HUS)?

Dysentery, renal failure, microangiopathic hemolytic anemia, thrombocytopenia

What causes it?

A shiga-like toxin produced by the *E. coli* O157:H7 strain, which has been linked to contaminated foods (animal feces)

What patient populations are typically affected?

Children and elderly

How is it treated?

Supportive measures. Avoid antibiotics and antimotility agents (use in HUS has been associated with increased morbidity and mortality)

What is the differential diagnosis of chronic diarrhea in an HIV patient?

Protozoal infection, MAC, CMV colitis, HIV colitis, highly active antiretroviral therapy (HAART)-related

What is the name for the infection caused by *C. difficile*?

Pseudomembranous colitis

When is the intestinal tract most susceptible to overcolonization with *C. difficile*?

After alteration of normal gut flora by antibiotics or chemotherapy, classically clindamycin

What does *C. difficile* toxin cause?

Secretory or bloody diarrhea and an inflammatory response

How is *C. difficile* typically diagnosed?

Identification of *C. difficile* toxin in stool and pseudomembranes on colonoscopy

How is it treated?

Cessation of implicated antibiotic. Metronidazole is the drug of choice for treatment, but vancomycin given orally is an alternative

Using alcohol-based antibacterial hand gels will kill *C. difficile*. True or false?

False. You must wash your hands with soap and water.

What is the diagnosis when a patient presents with chronic abdominal pain, altered bowel habit (diarrhea or constipation), and abdominal bloating, but with no identifiable structural or biochemical disorder?

Irritable bowel syndrome (IBS)

What class of medications can be helpful in reducing the symptoms of IBS compared with placebo in the short term?

Antidepressants (amitriptyline, clomipramine, desipramine, doxepin, mianserin, trimipramine)

INFLAMMATORY BOWEL DISEASE

What two diseases are classified as inflammatory bowel disease (IBD)?

1. Ulcerative colitis (UC)
2. Crohn disease

What layer(s) of the colon wall are inflamed in UC?

Mucosal layer only

What layer(s) of the colon wall are inflamed in Crohn disease?

All layers (transmural)

What portions of the GI tract are affected by UC?

UC affects the rectum and may extend and involve the proximal colon

What portions of the GI tract are affected by Crohn disease?

Any portion of the entire GI tract from mouth to anus (80% involve the distal ileum)

What are the risk factors for IBD?

Caucasian or Jewish ethnicity, age between 15 and 30 and 50 and 70 (bimodal age distribution), female gender (for Crohn disease) and male gender (for UC), family history of IBD, cigarette smoking (for Crohn disease)

What genetic association does UC have?

HLA DR2

What are the typical symptoms of UC?

Bloody diarrhea with mucus passage and abdominal pain, possibly with tenesmus, fever, and weight loss

What are the typical symptoms of Crohn disease?

Prolonged history of diarrhea; crampy abdominal pain; fatigue; weight loss, with or without gross bleeding

What is the name for the complication commonly seen in Crohn disease when inflammation results in impaired colonic motility, colonic dilation, and decreased frequency of bowel movements?

Toxic megacolon

   What class of medications may precipitate it?

Antidiarrheals

   How does the patient present?

High fever, leukocytosis, abdominal tenderness, rebound tenderness, dilated segment of colon on abdominal XR

   How is it treated?

Bowel rest; nasogastric tube; IV fluids; antibiotics to cover GI flora; steroids, if the cause is IBD

What are the gastrointestinal complications of Crohn disease?

Bowel perforation, fibrotic strictures with bowel obstruction, abscess formation, fistula formation, anal fissures, perirectal abscesses, aphthous ulcers, dysphagia

What are the extraintestinal complications of IBD?

Uveitis, episcleritis, erythema nodosum, pyoderma gangrenosum, peripheral arthritis, ankylosing spondylitis, sclerosing cholangitis, venous thromboembolism

What endoscopic findings are consistent with a diagnosis of UC?

Continuous involvement of the colon, varying in severity from erythematous mucosa with petechiae and friability to macroulcerations and profuse bleeding

What biopsy findings are characteristic of UC?

Crypt abscesses and chronic changes, such as atrophied glands and lost mucin in goblet cells

What endoscopic findings are consistent with a diagnosis of Crohn disease?

Skip lesions, with focal ulcerations adjacent to normal mucosa, and a "cobblestone" appearance of polypoid mucosal changes

What biopsy findings are characteristic of Crohn disease?

Focal ulcerations with both acute and chronic inflammation, noncaseating granulomas

What features distinguish the diagnosis of colon-involving Crohn disease from ulcerative colitis?

Rectal sparing, coinvolvement of the small bowel, lack of gross bleeding, perianal involvement, fistula formation, granuloma presence, focal lesions

What medication is considered first-line therapy in IBD?

5-aminosalicylate (5-ASA) containing compounds

What 5-ASA containing medication can be used for UC or Crohn disease limited to the colon?

Sulfasalazine (metabolized to 5-ASA in the colon)

What 5-ASA containing medication can be used for Crohn disease involving the small bowel?

Mesalamine

What autoantibodies have been classically associated with IBD?

P-ANCA (UC), ASCA (Crohn disease)

What class of medications is used to induce remission in flare-ups of moderate to severe disease, treat extraintestinal manifestations or when 5-ASA medications do not work?

Glucocorticoids

What medications can be used for refractory cases of IBD?

Immunomodulating medications, such as 6-mercaptopurine, azathioprine, methotrexate, cyclosporine, and infliximab

When should surgery be considered for IBD?

Life-threatening bleeding, fistulas, obstruction, perforation, abscesses, and in medically refractory disease or neoplastic transformation

Is the risk for colorectal cancer higher for Crohn or UC?

UC

CHAPTER 22

Blood in Stool

What are the common causes of lower GI bleeding in newborns?	Swallowed maternal blood, anorectal fissures, necrotizing enterocolitis, malrotation with volvulus, Hirschsprung disease, coagulopathy
What diagnosis should you suspect in an infant with nonspecific systemic signs, such as apnea, respiratory failure, lethargy, poor feeding, abdominal distention, vomiting, or diarrhea?	Necrotizing enterocolitis (NEC)
What is the hallmark radiographic finding?	Pneumatosis intestinalis, gas bubbles in the bowel wall
What is the major risk factor for this condition?	Prematurity
An infant presents with abdominal distension, bilious emesis, and melena. What is your diagnosis?	Malrotation with midgut volvulus
What are the common causes of GI bleeding in infants?	Allergic colitis, intussusception, Meckel diverticulum, Henoch-Schonlein purpura, hemolytic uremic syndrome, lymphonodular hyperplasia
What are the classic exam findings in an infant with intussusception?	Currant-jelly stools, mass in abdomen, vomiting
What is the diagnostic test of choice?	Ultrasonography or contrast enema
Guaiac positive stools, cutaneous purpura over buttocks and lower extremities, swelling of feet and joint pains in a child suggest what diagnosis?	Henoch-Schonelin purpura

What test can be used to differentiate fetal from maternal blood?

Apt test

What are the two major causes of iron deficiency in developed countries?

1. GI blood loss
2. Menstrual blood loss in women

What is the differential diagnosis of occult GI bleeding?

Colon CA, esophagitis, peptic ulcer disease, gastritis, IBD, vascular ectasias, diverticula, celiac disease, portal hypertensive gastropathy

The presence of occult GI bleeding, epistaxis, and oral telangiectasias suggests what hereditary syndrome?

Osler-Weber-Rendu syndrome (also known as HHT: hereditary hemorrhagic telangiectasia)

False positive occult blood tests can result from ingestion of what?

Red meat, dietary peroxidases (such as turnips and radishes)

False negative results on occult blood tests can result from ingestion of what vitamin?

Vitamin C

Minimal bright red bleeding per rectum (BRBPR), or "outlet bleeding" includes what complaints?

Small amounts of blood on toilet paper after wiping, few drops of blood in toilet bowl, or small amounts of blood on surface of stool

The following histories in additional to minimal BRBPR suggest what conditions?

    Painless bleeding with defecation

Internal hemorrhoids

    Sharp pain with bowel movements

Anal fissure, rectal CA, herpes, recent anal trauma, or instrumentation

    Intermittent rectal bleeding, passage of mucus, mild diarrhea

Proctitis

    Passage of mucus, straining with defecation, and sense of incomplete evacuation

Rectal ulcer

    Abdominal pain, change in bowel habits

Colon cancer

Maroon stool with intermixed bright red blood (hematochezia) implies bleeding from what part of the GI tract?

Proximal colon or small intestine

What test can be done in a patient with hematochezia to rule out an upper GI source proximal to the ligament of Treitz?

Nasogastric tube lavage or endoscopy

A history of melena and/or hematemesis suggests bleeding from what source?

Upper GI or slow proximal colon bleeding

What are important things to ask for in the history of a patient with rectal bleeding?

Age, systemic symptoms, change in frequency or caliber of stools, history of inflammatory bowel disease, family history of colon cancer, history of anal trauma, history of pelvic radiation

What physical exam is required in the evaluation of rectal bleeding?

External inspection of anus, digital rectal exam, fecal occult blood testing, office-based anoscopy or proctoscopy

What special measures should you take in a person with ongoing rectal bleeding, transfusion requirement greater than two units of packed red blood cells, or signs of hemodynamic instability?

Admit to ICU, start two large caliber peripheral catheters or central venous line

An elderly patient presents with left-sided abdominal pain and rectal bleeding after a recent episode of hypotension after surgery. What is your likely diagnosis?

Ischemic colitis

What are indications for additional testing in a patient with BRBPR regardless of age?

Vital sign abnormalities, constitutional symptoms, change in frequency of stools, anemia, melena, fecal occult blood positive stools, family history of familial polyposis

What is the diagnostic test indicated when you cannot find a cause for rectal bleeding in a patient under age 50?

Sigmoidoscopy or colonoscopy

What is the diagnostic test indicated identified for ANY rectal bleeding in a patient OVER age 50?

Colonoscopy

What is the recommended evaluation for a patient with occult GI bleeding and anemia or upper GI symptoms?

Upper endoscopy and colonoscopy

When should you consider endoscopic evaluation in a premenopausal woman with anemia?	Positive fecal occult blood test, anemia out of proportion to menstrual blood loss, family history of early GI malignancy
What is the grading of internal hemorrhoids?	Grade 1: no prolapse. Grade 2: prolapse with defecation, but reduce spontaneously. Grade 3: prolapse with defecation, require manual reduction. Grade 4: prolapsed and cannot be reduced manually.
What is the initial treatment for bleeding and grade 1 or 2 hemorrhoids?	Adding fiber to diet or using fiber supplement with psyllium or methylcellulose, ensuring adequate fluid intake
What is the best initial treatment for irritation and pruritus associated with hemorrhoids?	Warm sitz baths, hydrocortisone suppositories, analgesic creams
What is the treatment of acute thrombosed external hemorrhoids not improving within 24 to 48 hours?	Surgical evacuation of hemorrhoid with excision of skin overlying it
What are the nonsurgical treatment options for grade 1-3 internal hemorrhoids refractory to conservative therapy?	Rubber band ligation, infrared coagulation, laser photocoagulation, sclerotherapy, cryosurgery, and bipolar diathermy (Bicap)
Operative therapy is indicated for hemorrhoids with what characteristics?	Failure of medical and nonoperative therapy, concomitant anorectal condition requiring surgery, symptomatic third-degree, fourth-degree, or mixed internal and external hemorrhoids

DIVERTICULAR DISEASE

What are diverticula?	Sac-like protrusions of the colon wall
What is the difference between diverticulosis and diverticulitis?	Diverticulosis describes the presence of diverticula, while diverticulitis is inflammation of those diverticula.
What is the prevalence of diverticular disease?	Less than 5% at age 40, 65% at age 85

Of individuals with diverticulosis, what percent:

Are asymptomatic	70%
Develop diverticulitis	20%
Develop diverticular bleeding	10%

What causes diverticular bleeding?

A penetrating arterial vessel becomes draped over a diverticulum as it forms (with only mucosa separating the vessel from the lumen, and the vasa recta ruptures into the lumen).

Diverticular bleeding is painful. True or false?

False. It is painless and usually self-limited.

Why are the diverticuli called false diverticula?

They don't contain all the layers of the colonic wall (mucosa and submucosa herniate through the muscle layer and are covered only by serosa)

Where do diverticula develop?

At points of weakness, where the vasa recta penetrates the circular muscle layer

Where in the colon do patients tend to get diverticula?

95% are sigmoid diverticula, 35% have disease proximal to the sigmoid

What is thought to cause diverticula?

Increased colon pressure by enhanced peristaltic contractions and a low-fiber diet

What causes diverticulitis?

Micro-perforation of diverticula by increased intraluminal pressure or inspissated food particles, resulting in inflammation and focal necrosis

What are the classic symptoms of diverticulitis?

Left lower quadrant (LLQ) pain, with or without nausea and vomiting; constipation; diarrhea; irritative urinary symptoms

What are the physical exam findings suggestive of diverticulitis?

LLQ tenderness; abdominal distention; tender, palpable mass; low-grade fever

What are the key lab findings in diverticulitis?

Mild leukocytosis, normal LFTs, sterile pyuria

What are the key CT findings in diverticulitis?

Increased soft tissue density within pericolic fat, colonic diverticula, bowel wall thickening

What are the complications of diverticulitis?

Abscess, peritonitis, fistula, obstruction, perforation

How should you manage uncomplicated acute diverticulitis?

Bowel rest, hydration, antibiotics (cover gram-negative rods and anaerobes)

What dietary recommendations are made for patients with diverticular disease?

High-fiber diet

How should you follow up a first episode of uncomplicated acute diverticulitis?

Colonoscopy or flexible sigmoidoscopy plus barium enema 2-6 weeks after resolution to rule out cancer and determine extent of disease

What are the indications for surgical intervention in diverticulitis?

Perforation, obstruction, abscess

COLORECTAL CANCER (CRC)

In the United States, what is the third leading cause of cancer and cancer death in men and women?

CRC

What are risk factors for CRC?

Age >40-50 years, personal history of CRC, personal history of polyps, first-degree relative diagnosed with CRC, IBD, cigarette smoking

In most cases of CRC, there is a positive family history of the disease. True or false?

False

What is familial adenomatous polyposis (FAP)?

A familial colon cancer syndrome in which a germline mutation in the adenomatous polyposis coli (APC) gene results in numerous colonic adenomas appearing during childhood

What percent of patients with FAP develop colon cancer?

90% by age 45

What is Lynch syndrome/HNPCC (hereditary nonpolyposis colorectal cancer)?

A familial colon cancer syndrome associated with defects in DNA mismatch repair

What genetic disorders predispose a person to CRC?

FAP, Gardner syndrome, HNPCC/Lynch syndrome

What is the most common presenting symptom of CRC?

Abdominal pain

What other symptoms may help localize the lesion to the

    Right side?

Iron-deficiency anemia, weight loss, anorexia

    Left side?

Decreased stool caliber, constipation, obstipation, diarrhea

    Rectum?

Bright red blood per rectum and/or tenesmus

What is the diagnostic test of choice for patients with symptoms suggestive of CRC?

Colonoscopy

    What if the colonoscope cannot reach the tumor site?

Double-contrast barium enema

What is the differential diagnosis of CRC?

Other malignancies (lymphoma, carcinoid, Kaposi sarcoma, or metastases), hemorrhoids, IBD, diverticulitis, infection

What are the most common sites of metastases of CRC?

Regional lymph nodes, liver, lungs, peritoneum

Can carcinoembryonic antigen (CEA) be used as a screening test for CRC?

No

When do you use CEA?

In patients newly diagnosed with CRC for both prognosis and evaluation

What does the metastatic workup of CRC involve?

CXR, LFTs, abdominal CT

What is the most important prognostic factor in CRC?

Depth of bowel wall invasion

What is the only curative modality for localized CRC?

Surgical resection

For average-risk individuals, at what age should CRC screening begin?

50 years

What are the different options for CRC screening?

Annual fecal occult blood test (FOBT), flexible sigmoidoscopy alone every 5 years, flexible sigmoidoscopy every 5 years with FOBT yearly, colonoscopy every 10 years

Which of the above has the greatest sensitivity and specificity?

Colonoscopy

What are some disadvantages to colonoscopy?

Risk of bleeding/perforation, patient has to do bowel prep, costly, sedation leads to longer recovery time (and adds indirect costs for transportation, absenteeism, etc)

What are some advantages to colonoscopy versus other types of screening?

Ability to localize lesions throughout the entire colon, biopsy mass lesions, and remove polyps

How should you screen patients with a family history of first-degree relative with CRC?

Colonoscopy every 10 years starting at age 40, or colonoscopy 10 years prior to the age at diagnosis of the youngest family member with CRC, whichever comes first

When should you start screening in a patient with inflammatory bowel disease?

Colonoscopy every 1-2 years starting 8-10 years after diagnosis, or 15 years after diagnosis, if disease is limited to the left colon

CHAPTER 23

Erectile Dysfunction

ERECTILE DYSFUNCTION

Male sexual dysfunction can be grouped into which categories?

Erectile dysfunction (ED), decreased libido, and ejaculation problems (retrograde ejaculation and premature ejaculation)

What is the definition of ED?

The inability to initiate or maintain an erection sufficient for satisfactory sexual performance

What is the prevalence of ED?

One-third of men at age 40 and two-thirds of men by the age of 70

What are common etiologies of ED?

Psychologic (anxiety, depression, life stressors), neurologic (diabetes, status postprostatectomy), endocrine (hypogonadism, hyperprolactinemia, thyroid disease), vascular (inadequate arterial flow into the corpora cavernosa from atherosclerosis), anatomic (Peyronie disease leading to fibrous plaques involving the corpora cavernosa)

What medications can cause ED?

Antihypertensives (thiazides, spironolactone, beta-blockers, alpha-blockers), psychiatric medications (tri-cyclic antidepressants, monoamine oxidase inhibitors, selective serotonin reuptake inhibitors), alcohol, H2 antagonists (due to antiandrogenic properties)

What labs can be ordered to evaluate ED?

Serum total testosterone (drawn at the 8 AM testosterone peak to evaluate for hypogonadism), prolactin (elevated prolactin from a prolactinoma inhibits gonadotropin-releasing hormone [GnRH]), thyroid stimulation hormone (both hypo- and hyperthyroidism can contribute to ED), glucose and cholesterol (diabetes and hyperlipidemia are risk factors for arterial disease)

What are the first-line treatments for ED?

Phosphodiesterase-5 (PDE-5) inhibitors, psychotherapy (for anxiety or depression), testosterone replacement (for hypogonadism)

How do PDE-5 inhibitors work?

During an erection, intracavernosal cyclic GMP causes vasodilation and is broken down by PDE-5. PDE-5 inhibitors prevent the breakdown of cGMP.

What are the side effects of PDE-5 inhibitors?

The vasodilation can cause severe hypotension (when used in conjunction with nitrates), flushing, rhinitis, and lightheadedness.

What percentage of patients taking PDE-5 inhibitors will have priapism?

Less than 2%. Patients with erections lasting more than 4 hours should seek immediate medical assistance.

What is the duration of action of PDE-5 inhibitors?

Sildenafil and vardenafil start working 30 minutes after ingestion and last for 4 hours. Absorption of these two medications is decreased with high fat meals. Tadalafil starts working 16 minutes after ingestion and lasts for 36 hours.

What treatments can be tried after failure of first-line treatments for ED?

Intrapenile injections, intraurethral alprostadil, vacuum pumps, semirigid or inflatable prostheses

What treatment can be offered to men with ED secondary to hypogonadism?

Testosterone replacement (commonly delivered using a patch or gel)

What are the side effects of testosterone replacement?

Increased prostate volume, erythrocytosis, skin irritation from transdermal testosterone, increased sleep apnea symptoms, hyperlipidemia

CHAPTER 24

Scrotal Pain and Swelling

SCROTAL PAIN AND SWELLING

What conditions can cause scrotal pain?

Testicular torsion, torsion of the appendix testis or epididymis, epididymitis, incarcerated inguinal hernia, Henoch-Schonlein purpura, orchitis

What conditions can cause scrotal swelling or a scrotal mass?

Hydrocele, varicocele, nonincarcerated inguinal hernia, spermatocele, nephrotic syndrome, testicular cancer, sperm granuloma (postvasectomy)

TESTICULAR TORSION

What is the bell clapper deformity?

A deformity where the testicle lacks a normal attachment to the tunica vaginalis. If the lower pole of the testis is inadequately attached to the tunica vaginalis, the testis may twist on the spermatic cord.

What is the incidence of testicular torsion?

1 in 4000 in males younger than 25 years old (there is a small peak in the neonatal period and a large one in puberty though torsion can occur at any age)

Why is testicular torsion seen more commonly in adolescence?

The increased incidence is thought to be from the increasing weight of testes during puberty.

What signs and symptoms are seen with testicular torsion?

Sudden onset of testicular or scrotal pain (can awaken the patient at night); pain is constant unless the testicle is intermittently detorsing; vomiting; scrotal edema, tenderness, and elevation (due to cord shortening); absent cremasteric reflex; horizontally lying testis

What is a normal cremasteric reflex?

Upon scratching the upper, medial thigh, the ipsilateral testis elevates (absent before 30 months of age and typically unreliable in patients older than 12 years of age)

How is testicular torsion diagnosed?

Can be diagnosed clinically or by Doppler ultrasound (will show decreased testicular flow) or a nuclear scan of the scrotum (if the diagnosis is still uncertain)

How is testicular torsion treated?

Urgent consultation with urology, surgical detorsion and orchiopexy of both testes

What percentage of testes are viable after 12 hours of torsion?

20% (0% is viable after 24 hours)

TORSION OF THE APPENDIX TESTIS OR APPENDIX EPIDIDYMIS

What is the appendix testis?

A vestigial structure located on the anterosuperior aspect of the testis (present in 90%)

What is the appendix epididymis?

A vestigial structure located at the head of the epididymis (present in 23%)

Which patients are typically affected by torsion of these structures?

7-12 year olds

What signs and symptoms are seen with torsion of these structures?	Sudden onset of scrotal pain (typically less intense than testicular torsion), tender localized testicular or epididymal mass, blue dot sign (the appendix has become gangrenous), normal cremasteric reflex
How is this condition diagnosed?	Can be diagnosed clinically, although Doppler ultrasound can be used when testicular torsion cannot be excluded
How is it managed?	Analgesics, scrotal support, reassurance (symptoms resolve in 5-10 days), surgery for patients with persistent pain

EPIDIDYMITIS

What are the signs and symptoms of acute bacterial epididymitis?	Dysuria, frequency, urgency, testicular pain, fever
What are the causative organisms in infectious epididymitis in males below 35 years of age?	*Chlamydia trachomatis* (most common), *Neisseria gonorrhoeae*
What are the causative organisms in infectious epididymitis in males over 35 years of age?	*Escherichia coli, Pseudomonas,* sexually transmitted organisms are possible, but less common
What is the pathogenesis of noninfectious epididymitis?	Urine refluxes through the ejaculatory ducts and vas deferens into the epididymis resulting in chemical inflammation
What are the risk factors for noninfectious epididymitis?	Prolonged sitting, vigorous exercise (heavy lifting)
What is Prehn sign?	Decreased pain with scrotal elevation, suggesting the patient has epididymitis rather than testicular torsion
Is Prehn sign a reliable way of diagnosing epididymitis?	No. It also does not reliably exclude testicular torsion.

What are the treatments for infectious epididymitis?	Ice, scrotal elevation/support, NSAIDs, if <35 years, then ceftriaxone 250 mg IM × 1 day and doxycycline 100 mg PO BID × 10 days, if >35 years, then ofloxacin 300 mg PO BID × 10 days or levofloxacin 500 mg PO QD × 10 days

HYDROCELE

What is a hydrocele?	Peritoneal fluid collecting between the parietal and visceral layers of the tunica vaginalis
How are communicating hydroceles different from noncommunicating hydroceles?	Noncommunicating hydroceles do not communicate with the peritoneal cavity, are not reducible, and do not change in size with Valsalva
What conditions can cause secondary noncommunicating hydroceles?	Epididymitis, orchitis, testicular torsion, trauma, testicular cancer
When should you order an ultrasound to evaluate a hydrocele?	When you suspect that the hydrocele is secondary
Do hydroceles transilluminate?	Yes
What are the indications for surgery for hydroceles?	Newborns with hydroceles that persist past one year of age; communicating hydroceles, since they increase the risk of the development of incarcerated inguinal hernias; symptomatic hydroceles

VARICOCELE

What are varicoceles?	Dilated veins in the pampiniform plexus from increased venous pressure and incompetent valves

On which side are varicoceles typically seen?	90% occur on the left side because the left spermatic vein enters the left renal vein at a 90° angle while the right spermatic vein enters the inferior vena cava (IVC) more obtusely allowing for smoother flow
What percentage of males with varicoceles will develop fertility problems?	10%-15%
What signs are seen with varicoceles?	Varicoceles feel like a "bag of worms," enlarge with Valsalva, and typically decrease when the patient is supine
When should you be concerned about a secondary varicocele?	Persists in the supine position, acute onset, right sided
What conditions can cause secondary varicoceles?	IVC thrombus, right renal vein thrombus, abdominal mass (retroperitoneal tumor or kidney tumor)

INGUINAL HERNIA

What is the lifetime risk of developing a groin hernia (inguinal or femoral)?	25% in males and 5% in females
How do indirect inguinal hernias develop?	The hernia comes from the internal ring where the spermatic cord (in males) and the round ligament (in females) exits the abdomen. The failure of the internal ring to close (following migration of the testicle into the inguinal canal) combined with the failure of obliteration of the processus vaginalis lead to the defect through which the hernia can develop.
On which side do indirect hernias frequently develop?	The right, which is the side that descends last
The origin of indirect inguinal hernias is lateral to the inferior epigastric artery. True or false?	True. Direct inguinal hernias are medial to the inferior epigastric artery.

How do direct inguinal hernias develop?

Direct inguinal hernias develop through Hesselbach triangle (formed by the inguinal ligament inferiorly, the inferior epigastric vessels laterally, and the rectus abdominis muscle medially). These hernias are the result of weakness (which can be congenital or acquired) in the floor of the inguinal canal.

What are the clinical manifestations of inguinal hernias?

Inguinal hernias cause heaviness or dull discomfort in the inguinal region that is increased with straining or lifting and relieved by lying down. The discomfort is often worse at the end of the day after prolonged standing. Patients can also be asymptomatic.

List the steps in evaluating a patient with a suspected hernia.

Visually inspect the patient in the standing position. Using the second or third finger, invaginate the scrotal skin and follow the spermatic cord upward to the triangular opening of the external inguinal canal. If possible, follow the inguinal canal laterally. With your finger in the external ring or within the canal, ask the patient to cough. Note any mass as it touches your finger.

What is an incarcerated hernia?

A hernia that cannot be manually reduced

What happens when an incarcerated hernia becomes strangulated?

There is decreased blood flow to the contents of an incarcerated hernia leading to ischemia and necrosis.

Why are inguinal hernia repairs performed?

Inguinal hernia repairs are performed to reduce symptoms and prevent hernia strangulation. Watchful waiting is an acceptable option for asymptomatic, minimal hernias in patients who wish to avoid surgery.

TESTICULAR CANCER

Testicular cancer represents what percentage of cancers in males aged 15-35?

20% (it is the most common solid tumor in this age group)

What are the two tumor cell types associated with 90% of testicular cancers?

1. Seminoma
2. Nonseminomatous germ cell (choriocarcinoma, embryonal, teratoma, yolk sac)

Cryptorchidism increases the risk of testicular cancer. True or false?

True. Cryptorchidism increases the risk 40 fold.

What are signs and symptoms of testicular cancer?

Painless, firm testicular mass; mass does not transilluminate (although a reactive hydrocele can be present); some patients have gynecomastia

If testicular cancer is suspected, what imaging tests should be ordered?

Scrotal ultrasound (an MRI can help if the ultrasound is inconclusive)

What is the USPSTF recommendation regarding routine screening for testicular cancer in asymptomatic adolescent and adult males?

D—it recommends against routine screening

What tumor markers should be collected in a patient with suspected testicular cancer?

Complete blood count, beta subunit of human chorionic gonadotropin (beta-hCG), alpha fetoprotein (AFP), lactate dehydrogenase (LDH)

CHAPTER 25

Urinary Incontinence and Retention

URODYNAMIC TESTING

What is urodynamic testing?

A study that measures the properties of the structures required for urination

What quantitative measurements does it take?

Urine volume and flow rate, bladder volume capacity, bladder and rectal pressure at various bladder volumes and during urination, pressure at which urine leakage occurs, postvoid residual, nerve impulses, and muscle activity around urethral sphincter

What urinary symptoms does it help evaluate?

Frequency, urgency, incontinence, hesitancy, retention, dysuria, recurrent urinary tract infections

INCONTINENCE

What is urinary incontinence?

Involuntary loss of urine

What are the types of urinary incontinence?

Stress incontinence, urge incontinence, neuropathic incontinence (overflow), mixed incontinence

What is stress incontinence?

Involuntary loss of urine when the intraabdominal pressure (created by coughing, lifting, sneezing) is greater than the pressure generated by the urinary sphincter

What patient population is most commonly affected by stress incontinence?

Middle-aged, multiparous women

What is the underlying pathophysiology of stress incontinence?

Weakness of the pelvic floor and hypermobility of the vesicourethral segment

What is a Marshall test and when is it positive?

With a full bladder, a woman lies on her back with her knees bent and feet in stirrups (dorsal lithotomy), then the examiner observes the urethral meatus when the patient coughs. If urine leaks, the test is positive and indicates pelvic floor instability.

What is the definitive treatment for stress incontinence?

Surgical pelvic floor suspension

What other nonpharmacologic therapy can help stress incontinence?

Mild cases can respond to Kegel exercises to strengthen the pelvic floor musculature or the use of pessaries in females

What is urge incontinence?

Incontinence due to detrusor muscle spasms acting against a functioning urinary sphincter resulting in a sudden urge to urinate

What are the common signs of urge incontinence?

No findings on physical examination, but urodynamic studies will detect abnormality

What medications are used to treat urge incontinence?

Anticholinergic medications (oxybutynin, tolterodine) to prevent detrusor spasm

What are the common side effects of anticholinergic medications?

Dry mouth, dizziness, drowsiness, urinary retention, constipation, nausea, blurry vision

What is an absolute contraindication to anticholinergic therapy?

Uncontrolled narrow angle glaucoma

| What is neuropathic incontinence? | Incontinence caused by a lesion of the nervous system (stroke, spinal cord lesion, dementia) |
| What is the treatment for neuropathic incontinence? | Intermittent self-catheterization |

CYSTOCELES AND OTHER PELVIC FLOOR ABNORMALITIES

What is a cystocele?	A hernia in which the urinary bladder protrudes through the wall of the vagina
What are the urinary symptoms of a cystocele?	Stress incontinence or incomplete voiding
What causes a cystocele?	Significant or repeated exertion (heavy lifting, childbirth, straining with bowel movement) creating increased abdominal pressure, sometimes accompanied by a decrease in estrogen (keeps pelvic floor muscles strong)
Because many of their causes overlap, cystoceles often occur together with enteroceles, urethroceles, and rectoceles. Describe each one of these.	
Enteroceles	Protrusion of bowel into the vaginal canal, which may occur after hysterectomy. May cause lower back pain
Urethroceles	Protrusion of urethra into vaginal canal. May cause incontinence
Rectocele	The front part of the rectum bulges into the vagina. May cause dyspareunia, constipation, and incomplete defecation. Patients sometimes need to use manual pressure against posterior vaginal wall or perineum in order to defecate.

These pelvic floor abnormalities are graded by their degree of protrusion relative to the vaginal introitus (vaginal opening). Describe the three grades.

| Grade I | Protrusion that does not reach the introitus |

Grade II — Protrusion reaches introitus

Grade III — Protrusion goes beyond introitus

What is uterine prolapse?

Descent of the uterus from its normal position into the vaginal canal causing discomfort and pain, dyspareunia, incontinence, and recurring urogenital infections

What physical exam maneuvers allow visualization of pelvic floor defects?

A single blade speculum is used to apply pressure to the vaginal wall. Posterior defects are seen with pressure applied to the anterior wall. Anterior defects are seen with pressure applied to the posterior wall. Sometimes the patient has to Valsalva or stand up to make the abnormality detectable.

What is a pessary?

A device inserted in the vagina that is used to support the vagina, uterus, bladder, and or rectum. It is used to treat pelvic floor defects.

What is the definitive treatment of pelvic floor defects?

Surgery

URINARY RETENTION

What is urinary retention?

The inability to voluntarily urinate, usually accompanied by intense discomfort

What is a postvoid residual (PVR) and how is it typically measured?

PVR is the amount of urine left in the bladder after urination. It may be measured with a bladder scan (pelvic ultrasound) or catheter and done alone or in conjunction with other urodynamic testing.

A measurement of how many milliliters or more is an abnormal PVR?	100 mL
What causes of urinary retention are seen in both men and women?	Obstruction (calculi, mass, fecal impaction, strictures, contractures, foreign bodies, edema, abscess), urogenital infection or inflammation (herpes simplex, cystitis), neurogenic bladder (transverse myelitis, spinal surgery, stroke), urogenital trauma, psychologic disturbance
What causes urinary retention in men?	Penile pathology causing obstruction, inflammation, and/or pain (balanitis, meatal stenosis, phimosis, constricting bands); prostate disease (benign prostatic hyperplasia, prostate cancer, prostatitis)
What is the most common cause of urinary retention in men?	Benign prostatic hyperplasia (BPH)
What causes urinary retention in women?	Organ prolapse (cystocele, rectocele, uterine prolapsed), gynecological masses (tumors, cysts), infectious or inflammatory vulvovaginal lesions (vaginal lichen planus, vaginal lichen sclerosis, vaginal pemphigus, herpes simplex), obstetrical complications
By what mechanism can infectious or inflammatory vulvovaginal lesions cause urinary retention?	Painful urination and urethral edema

PROSTATE CANCER

What cancer is the most common cancer in men and the second leading cause of cancer death in men?	Prostate cancer (CaP)
What are the risk factors for CaP?	Advanced age, positive family history, African American ethnicity, high dietary fat intake
How does CaP present?	Early disease may be asymptomatic but detectable by screening. Urinary obstruction symptoms, erectile dysfunction, and hematospermia are uncommon but more typical in advance disease.

What are the screening methods for CaP?

Digital rectal exam (DRE) and prostate specific antigen (PSA)

What DRE findings would suggest malignancy?

Hard and irregular nodules, usually in the peripheral zone (70%)

Besides CaP, what can cause a PSA elevation?

Benign prostatic hyperplasia, acute prostatitis, prostate massage, prostate biopsy, ejaculation, digital rectal examination, perineal trauma

What is the cutoff for identifying an elevated PSA that has been used in screening studies?

4 ng/mL

What is the sensitivity and specificity of using this cutoff to identify CaP?

Sensitivity of 70%-80%, specificity of 60%-70%

What are the potential harms from PSA screening?

Additional medical visits, adverse effects of prostate biopsies, anxiety, overdiagnosis (identifying prostate cancer that would never have caused symptoms during the patient's lifetime)

Have any high quality randomized controlled trials demonstrated that PSA screening decreases morbidity or mortality?

No. A Cochrane meta-analysis found no difference in CaP mortality between men invited to CaP screening and control groups. According to the USPSTF, there is insufficient data to determine whether PSA screening decreases morbidity or mortality.

How is a definitive diagnosis of CaP made?

Biopsy (ultrasound guided)

After lymph nodes, what is the most common site of CaP metastasis?

Bone

What is the most common symptom of bone metastasis?

Pain

BENIGN PROSTATIC HYPERPLASIA

What is benign prostatic hyperplasia (BPH)?	It is prostate enlargement that can cause symptoms of urinary obstruction (hesitancy, retention). Its prevalence increases with age, and it is considered a normal part of aging in men over the age of 50 years.
What area of the prostate does BPH most commonly occur?	Central zone
Is BPH always detectable on exam?	No
What are the obstructive symptoms of BPH?	Retention, hesitancy, decreased stream, sensation of incomplete voiding, straining, postvoid dribbling
What are the irritative symptoms of BPH?	Urgency, frequency, hematuria, nocturia
What digital DRE findings are characteristic of BPH?	Uniform enlargement, rubbery texture
In a patient with a history of BPH, what is the most likely cause of a palpable suprapubic mass and elevated creatinine?	Obstruction from BPH causing distended bladder (palpable suprapubic mass) and renal insufficiency (elevated creatinine)
According to the American Urological Association, is it necessary to measure PSA in BPH patients?	No. PSA measurement is usually optional. Follow PSA if the patient has a ≥10-year life expectancy, if knowledge of the presence of prostate cancer would change management, or if PSA measurement changes management of the patient's voiding symptoms.
What is the medical treatment of BPH?	Alpha-adrenergic blockers (prazosin, terazosin), 5-alpha reductase inhibitors (finasteride)
What is the mechanism of action of alpha-1-adrenergic blockers?	Relax the prostatic smooth muscle alleviating the dynamic component of the obstruction and relax the bladder's internal sphincter
What are the common side effects of alpha-1-adrenergic blockers?	Orthostatic hypotension, retrograde ejaculation

How long does it take these drugs to effect a change in symptoms?	1 week
What is the mechanism of action of 5-alpha reductase inhibitors?	Decrease the size of the prostate by inhibiting the conversion of testosterone to the more potent androgen dihydrotestosterone (DHT)
What are the common side effects of 5-alpha reductase inhibitors?	Decreased libido, decreased ejaculate volume, impotence, gynecomastia
What effect do 5-alpha reductase inhibitors have on PSA?	Reduce the PSA by 50%
How long does it take for 5-alpha reductase inhibitors to have their full effect?	6 months
What is the surgical treatment of BPH?	Transurethral resection of the prostate (TURP) or open prostatectomy, if severe
What are the indications for surgical intervention in BPH?	Refractory urinary retention, recurrent UTI from BPH, recurrent gross hematuria, bladder stone formation, renal failure, large bladder diverticula

CHAPTER 26

Dysuria and Vaginitis

DYSURIA

What is the definition of dysuria?

Pain, tingling, or burning just after urination

What is the differential diagnosis of dysuria in males?

Prostatitis, epididymitis, urethritis, urinary tract infection (UTI), primary herpes simplex infection

What is the differential diagnosis of dysuria in females?

UTI, urethritis, pyelonephritis, cervicitis, vaginitis, interstitial cystitis, primary herpes simplex infection

What cause of dysuria affects younger women and is characterized by urgency, small, frequent voids, and a normal urinalysis?

Interstitial cystitis

What are the treatment options for interstitial cystitis?

Oral pentosan polysulfate, intravesical dimethyl sulfoxide (DMSO), bladder training, tricyclic antidepressants

URINARY TRACT INFECTIONS

Lower UTIs include infections of which structures?

Urethra (urethritis), bladder (cystitis)

What are some of the common risk factors for UTI?

Sexual activity, diaphragm and spermicide use, previous UTI, catheters or urologic instrumentation, obstruction (BPH, stones, adhesions), pregnancy, diabetes, immunosuppression

How is the diagnosis of UTI established?

Characteristic clinical symptoms and urinalysis

When would you consider ordering a urine culture?

When there is an unclear diagnosis, a concern for antibiotic resistance, or a treatment failure

What are typical symptoms of UTIs?

Dysuria, frequency, urgency, suprapubic pain, and/or gross hematuria

What symptoms might you also see in a child with a UTI?

Bed-wetting, poor feeding, irritability, and/or fever

What etiology should you suspect in a child with recurrent UTIs?

Vesicoureteral reflux

What test do you order to evaluate this condition?

Voiding cystourethrogram (VCUG)

UTIs may cause several changes in the urine detectable by gross examination. What are some of these changes?

Cloudy urine, pungent odor, gross hematuria

UTIs present with what findings on urinalysis?

Pyuria, positive leukocyte esterase, positive urinary nitrite, hematuria, and/or proteinuria

What kinds of cells produce leukocyte esterase?

Neutrophils

When are nitrites found in the urine?

When organisms (many Gram-negative and some Gram-positive bacteria) that can reduce urinary nitrates to nitrites are present in significant numbers (at least 10,000 per mL)

A negative test for nitrites rules out a urinary tract infection. True or false?

False. A test for nitrites is very specific but not highly sensitive. However, keep in mind that air reacts with the dipstick reagent for nitrites and so the strips will produce false-positive results if overexposed to air.

What is the only group of persons that should be treated for asymptomatic bacteriuria?

Pregnant women

What are the most common UTI pathogens?

Escherichia coli (80%), *Staphylococcus saprophyticus* (4.4%), *Klebsiella pneumoniae* (4.3%), *Proteus mirabilis* (3.7%)

What organisms can cause urinary tract infections (as evidenced by pyuria) but produce negative urine cultures?

Viruses, tuberculosis, *Chlamydia*, *Ureaplasma urealyticum*

What are complicated UTIs?

UTIs that occur in patients who have conditions that increase the risk for treatment failure (functional/anatomic abnormalities, pregnancy, hospitalization, indwelling catheters)

What antibiotic regimens may be used as first-line treatment of an uncomplicated UTI?

Trimethoprim/sulfamethoxazole double-strength tablet (160 mg/800 mg) PO daily for 3 days, nitrofurantoin 100 mg twice daily for 5 days, cefpodoxime 100 mg twice daily for 3 days, ciprofloxacin 250 mg twice daily for 3 days

What antibiotic regimens may be used as first-line treatment of a complicated UTI?

Ciprofloxacin 500 mg twice daily or levofloxacin 500 mg once daily for 7-14 days

What recommendations would you make for a woman who has recurrent urinary tract infections?

Void after intercourse (though no randomized controlled trials have evaluated this practice), antimicrobial prophylaxis (eg, nitrofurantoin) daily or after intercourse, topical estrogen therapy in postmenopausal women, cranberry juice (150-750 mL daily)

PYELONEPHRITIS

What is pyelonephritis?

Inflammation of the kidney and renal pelvis

What percentage of women with dysuria in the outpatient setting will have pyelonephritis?

5%

What signs and symptoms are suggestive of pyelonephritis?	Fever (symptoms of pyelonephritis without fever should prompt an evaluation for an alternative diagnosis), chills, costovertebral angle tenderness, nausea, vomiting, abdominal/pelvic pain, lower UTI signs and symptoms (dysuria, frequency, urgency)
What is the most common etiology of UTI and pyelonephritis?	Ascending infection
How is the diagnosis of pyelonephritis made?	Clinical diagnosis supported by lab findings, such as pyuria or WBC casts
What is the only laboratory test that can immediately and specifically support the diagnosis of pyelonephritis?	White cell casts (sign of infection in the renal medulla)
Pain in the flank on deep percussion of the kidneys over the costovertebral angle is also known as what sign?	Lloyd sign
Are imaging studies, such as CT or ultrasound helpful in establishing the diagnosis of pyelonephritis?	No
What are the indications for hospitalization in pyelonephritis?	Inability to tolerate oral hydration and medications, noncompliance with medical treatment, pregnancy, intractable pain, area of high resistance to antibiotics
What classes of antibiotics are used to treat pyelonephritis?	Fluoroquinolones and third-generation cephalosporins

CERVICITIS

What are the infectious causes of cervicitis?	*Chlamydia trachomatis, Neisseria gonorrhoeae*, herpes simplex, *Trichomonas vaginalis*
What signs and symptoms are suggestive of cervicitis?	Dysuria, frequency, endocervical discharge, postcoital bleeding, dyspareunia, vulvovaginal irritation

How does cervicitis appear on speculum examination?	Cervical or urethral discharge, erythema, friable cervix
What is ectropion?	Eversion of columnar cervical epithelium over the external os, often caused by oral contraceptives and found in adolescents. It is a normal finding and may look similar but should not be mistaken for cervicitis.
How can you differentiate between dysuria from sexually transmitted infections (STIs) versus UTIs?	STI: nitrite negative, urine culture negative UTI: nitrite positive, hematuria, urine culture positive Both: pyuria, leukocyte esterase positive
What tests can be used to confirm the diagnosis of gonococcal and chlamydial cervicitis?	DNA amplification tests on urine or urethral discharge, culture on Thayer-Martin agar (for gonorrhea only)
Which STI is the most prevalent in the United States?	Chlamydia
How is chlamydial cervicitis treated?	Azithromycin 1 g PO × 1 or doxycycline 100 mg PO bid × 7 days
If a patient has gonorrhea, for which other STI should you empirically treat?	Chlamydia
How is gonococcal cervicitis treated?	Ceftriaxone 125 mg IM × 1 or cefixime 400 mg PO × 1 or cefpodoxime 400 mg PO × 1 PLUS empiric treatment for chlamydia

PELVIC INFLAMMATORY DISEASE

What is the definition of pelvic inflammatory disease (PID)?	Acute, usually polymicrobial, infection/inflammation of the upper genital tract in women, involving any or all of the uterus, oviducts, ovaries, and pelvic peritoneum
How does cervicitis lead to PID?	Through ascending infection by microorganisms

What are the most common organisms found to cause PID?

N. gonorrhoeae, C. trachomatis, Mycoplasma genitalium, anaerobic and facultative organisms (*Prevotella, E. coli, Haemophilus influenzae*, group B streptococcus)

What are some typical signs and symptoms of PID?

Lower abdominal pain (90%), mucopurulent cervical discharge (75%), fever (50%), rebound tenderness, urethritis, proctitis, chills, abnormal uterine bleeding

What are the minimal clinical criteria needed to diagnose PID?

Cervical motion tenderness or uterine or adnexal tenderness in the presence of lower abdominal or pelvic pain

What laboratory tests should you perform if you suspect PID in a patient?

Pregnancy test, microscopy of cervical or vaginal discharge, CBC, gonorrhea/chlamydia tests, urinalysis

What study should you perform if the patient appears acutely ill with a pelvic mass?

Pelvic ultrasound to rule out a tubo-ovarian abscess (TOA)

What are the sequelae of untreated PID?

Ectopic pregnancy, infertility, chronic pelvic pain, recurrent salpingitis

What is the name for the syndrome of perihepatitis that occurs in 10% of patients with PID caused by *N. gonorrhoeae* or *C. trachomatis*?

Fitz-Hugh-Curtis syndrome

Which patients should you hospitalize for treatment of PID?

Pregnant, adolescent, poorly compliant, immunodeficient, high fever, inability to tolerate oral medication due to nausea and vomiting, TOA, upper peritoneal signs, inadequate response to outpatient therapy after 48 hours, uncertain diagnosis

What are some recommended outpatient regimens for treatment of PID?

Ceftriaxone 250 mg intramuscularly (IM) × 1 + doxycycline 100 mg PO BID for 14 days, cefoxitin 2 g IM × 1 + probenecid 1 g PO × 1 + doxycycline 100 mg PO BID for 14 days, cefotaxime 1 g IM × 1 + doxycycline 100 mg PO BID for 14 days, treat partner(s) also

What medication would you add if you suspected PID with *T. vaginalis* or bacterial vaginosis, a pelvic abscess or history of gynecologic instrumentation in the past 3 weeks?

Metronidazole 500 mg PO BID for 14 days

HERPES SIMPLEX

What are the signs and symptoms of primary genital herpes simplex virus (HSV) infection?

Multiple, shallow, tender ulcers that may be vesicular; fever; headache; dysuria; tender lymphadenopathy

What is the mean duration of lesions in patients with primary genital HSV?

19 days

What is the mean duration of lesions in patients with nonprimary genital HSV lesions?

10 days

What percentage of patients with primary HSV will develop aseptic meningitis?

8%

The majority of patients with HSV-2 primary infection will experience recurrence. True or false?

True

What is the median number of HSV-2 recurrences per year?

Four

What is the median number of HSV-1 recurrences per year?

One

What other conditions can present with genital ulcers?

Primary syphilis (typically painless), chancroid (deep, purulent ulcer with painful, inguinal lymphadenopathy)

What tests can be used to confirm a diagnosis of genital HSV?

Testing of vesicular fluid can include viral culture, Tzanck smear (though this cannot distinguish between HSV-1 and HSV-2), polymerase chain reaction (particularly useful for asymptomatic HSV shedding), and direct fluorescent antibody testing

When do HSV antibodies form?

Several weeks after infection and persist indefinitely

What are the benefits of treating patients with primary HSV with oral antiviral agents?

Decreased duration and severity of the infection by days to weeks, decreased risk of complicated primary HSV infection

Which antiviral agents are typically used?

Either acyclovir 400 mg PO three times daily, famciclovir 250 mg PO three times daily, or valacyclovir 1000 mg PO twice daily can be used, and each for 7-10 days.

What is complicated HSV?

Primary HSV infection with aseptic meningitis, encephalitis, transverse myelitis, hepatitis, pneumonitis, or disseminated HSV

What other treatments can be offered to patients with dysuria secondary to ulcerations?

Analgesics, sitz baths

What are the treatment options for patients with recurrent genital HSV?

Chronic suppressive therapy, episodic therapy, or watchful waiting can be initiated depending on the frequency of episodes. Patients with six or more episodes per year are frequently on chronic suppressive therapy.

What regimens can be used for chronic suppressive therapy?

Acyclovir 400 mg PO twice daily, famciclovir 250 mg PO twice daily, valacyclovir 500 mg PO once daily

What regimens can be used for episodic therapy?

Acyclovir 800 mg PO three times daily for 2 days, famciclovir 1000 mg PO twice daily for 1 day, valacyclovir 500 mg PO twice daily for 3 days

VAGINITIS

What is vaginitis?

Vaginal inflammation

What are some typical symptoms of vaginitis?

Vaginal discharge, pruritus, irritation, burning, soreness, odor, dyspareunia, dysuria

What are noninfectious causes of vaginitis?

Atrophic vaginitis, reaction to allergens (eg, latex condoms and antifungal agents), chemical irritation (eg, spermicides and hygiene products)

What are the infectious causes of vaginitis?

Bacterial vaginosis (BV), vulvovaginal candidiasis, *Trichomonas vaginalis*

What is the normal vaginal pH of a woman of reproductive age?

4.0-4.5

From where should the vaginal pH sample be obtained?

The vaginal sidewall to avoid the posterior fornix (pooled blood, semen, and cervical mucus can increase the pH)

What common vaginal bacteria accounts for this acidic environment?

Lactobacilli produce lactic acid and hydrogen peroxide, and the acidity is hostile to the growth of pathogens and inhibits bacterial adherence to vaginal squamous epithelial cells.

Which causes of vaginitis present with an elevated vaginal pH?

BV, *Trichomonas*, atrophic vaginitis (decreased estrogen decreases *Lactobacilli*)

What medications or practices can alter the normal vaginal pH?

Antibiotics (can decrease *Lactobacilli* leading to increased pH), oral contraceptive pills, sexual activity (semen can increase pH), douching (may increase pH)

How does normal physiologic vaginal discharge in a reproductive age woman appear?

White or transparent, mostly odorless, less than 4 mL per 24 hours

What are some nonpathogenic causes of an increased amount of vaginal discharge?

Pregnancy, oral contraceptive pill use, ovulation

What are the most important tests to diagnose vaginitis?

Vaginal pH and microscopy (saline wet mount and 10% KOH preps)

What type of cells will you see on the saline (wet mount) prep with BV?

"Clue cells" (vaginal squamous epithelial cells covered with bacteria)

What type of smell will you notice with the KOH prep in BV?

Gardnerella produces amines causing a fishy smell, known as the "whiff test."

What are Amstel criteria for diagnosing BV?

1. Abnormal gray discharge (often "fishy" smelling)
2. Vaginal pH >4.5
3. Positive amine "whiff test"
4. Clue cells seen on microscopy

Note: three out of four criteria must be present to diagnose BV.

How do you treat BV?

Metronidazole (500 mg PO BID × 7 days) or clindamycin (topical 2% cream or 300 mg PO BID for 7 days); both are safe in pregnancy

How does vulvovaginal candidiasis present?

Odorless white, thick "cottage cheese" discharge, vulvar itching, burning, dyspareunia, dysuria

What are risk factors for vaginal candidiasis?

Antibiotics; diabetes mellitus; increased estrogen (eg, oral contraceptive pills and pregnancy) leading to increased glycogen, which increases adherence to epithelial cells; immunosuppression

What do you see on microscopy in candidiasis (albicans-species)?

Budding yeast cells and pseudohyphae on saline and KOH mounts

Why is KOH mount preferred over a saline mount?

KOH destroys other cellular elements.

How do you treat uncomplicated candidiasis?

Topical or oral azoles, commonly oral fluconazole (a single dose of 150 mg)

How do you treat severe candidiasis?

Give a second dose of oral fluconazole 3 days after first dose.

How do you treat recurrent candidiasis?

Daily oral fluconazole for 7-14 days, then weekly for 6 months

What is the best method for treating candidiasis in pregnancy?

Topical azole therapy for 7 days

What are the signs and symptoms of trichomoniasis?

Copious, thin, yellow-green discharge; pruritus; dysuria; irritation

How does *Trichomonas* appear under microscopy?	Motile trichomonads with four flagella on saline prep if checked less than 20 minutes after specimen obtained
How is *Trichomonas* spread?	Sexual contact
How do you treat *Trichomonas*?	Metronidazole (2 g PO × 1), treat sexual partner(s) also
Trichomonas can cause what complications of pregnancy?	Preterm delivery, premature rupture of membranes
What cause of dysuria should you consider in a postmenopausal woman with a normal urinalysis and negative urine culture?	Atrophic vaginitis
What is the treatment for atrophic vaginitis?	Intravaginal estrogens (creams, suppositories, or vaginal rings)

URETHRITIS IN MEN

What are the signs and symptoms of urethritis?	Urethral discharge and/or dysuria
Which pathogens can cause urethritis?	*N. gonorrhoeae, C. trachomatis, M. genitalium*, herpes simplex virus, *Trichomonas vaginalis, Ureaplasma urealyticum*
What is the most common cause of nongonococcal urethritis?	*C. trachomatis*
Describe the urethral discharge of nongonococcal urethritis.	Mucoid or watery
Describe the urethral discharge of gonococcal urethritis.	Copious and purulent
What percentage of nongonococcal urethritis are asymptomatic?	5%-10%
What percentage of gonococcal urethritis are asymptomatic?	Approximately 40%

Which features confirm urethritis?

Mucopurulent discharge, Gram stain of urethral secretions demonstrating >5 white blood cells per high power field, positive leukocyte esterase test, more than 10 white blood cells per high power field on urine sediment, cultures and nucleic acid amplification tests for *C. trachomatis* and *N. gonorrhoeae*

What is the treatment for nongonococcal urethritis?

Azithromycin 1 g PO × 1 or doxycycline 100 mg PO twice daily for 7 days

What is the treatment for gonococcal urethritis?

Ceftriaxone 125 mg IM × 1 or cefixime 400 mg PO × 1 or cefpodoxime 400 mg PO × 1

How long should patients and their sexual partners refrain from sexual contact to avoid reinfection?

Until the patient and his/her partner(s) have completed their courses of antibiotics and all symptoms have resolved

PROSTATITIS

What are the different types of prostatitis?

Acute bacterial, chronic bacterial, chronic nonbacterial

What are signs and symptoms of acute bacterial prostatitis?

Fever, chills, dysuria, obstructive symptoms (dribbling, hesitancy, retention), tender edematous prostate

How do you diagnose acute bacterial prostatitis?

Clinical signs and symptoms, frequently associated with pyuria, positive urine culture

What are the signs and symptoms of chronic bacterial prostatitis?

Frequency, dysuria, urgency, perineal discomfort, discomfort during ejaculation, deep pelvic pain, pain radiating to the back

How do you treat acute and chronic bacterial prostatitis?

Fluoroquinolones or trimethoprim-sulfamethoxazole (continue antibiotics for 4-6 weeks), NSAIDs

What causes chronic nonbacterial prostatitis?

The etiology is unclear. Specific bacteria, trauma, autoimmunity, neuropathic pain, increased prostate pressure, and psychologic factors have been hypothesized.

What are the clinical manifestations of chronic nonbacterial prostatitis?

Urinary frequency; dysuria; perineal pain; absence of urinary tract disease, active urethritis, urethral strictures, neurologic disease, or urogenital cancer

What therapies have been studied in the treatment of chronic nonbacterial prostatitis?

Quinolones, alpha-blockers, NSAIDs, 5 alpha-reductase inhibitors, and sitz baths have been researched, though none have consistently proven to be beneficial.

CHAPTER 27

Vaginal Bleeding and Dysmenorrhea

VAGINAL BLEEDING

In a normal ovulatory cycle,

Cycle length is between	24 and 35 days
Menses last for	2 to 7 days
Blood loss is less than	80 mL per cycle (5 tablespoons)

Define the following terms.

Menorrhagia	Excessive or prolonged bleeding that occurs at normal intervals, blood loss is greater than 80 mL per cycle, periods last for more than 7 days
Oligomenorrhea	Menstrual periods that occur at intervals greater than 35 days
Amenorrhea	Absence of bleeding for at least three usual cycles
Polymenorrhea	Bleeding that occurs at intervals less than 24 days
Menometrorrhagia	Bleeding at irregular intervals with heavy flow (>80 mL) or prolonged duration (>7 days)
Intermenstrual bleeding	Bleeding that occurs between menses
Postcoital bleeding	Vaginal bleeding within 24 hours of vaginal intercourse

What term is used to describe bleeding from the uterus that falls outside the normal ovulatory criteria?

Abnormal uterine bleeding (AUB). Physician visits for AUB commonly occur in the first 3 years following menarche or in the perimenopausal period.

Besides obtaining a detailed history and physical, what is the first step in evaluating AUB in a woman of childbearing age?

Determine pregnancy status

What are common causes of abnormal genital tract bleeding within the first 3 years following menarche?

Anovulation (due to hypothalamic immaturity), coagulopathies, stress (psychologic or exercise-induced), pregnancy, infection (such as cervicitis)

What are common causes of abnormal genital tract bleeding during the reproductive years?

Anovulation, pregnancy, cancer (eg, endometrial or cervical), polyps (endometrial or cervical), leiomyomas, adenomyosis (endometrium within the myometrium), infection (cervicitis, endometritis), endocrine dysfunction (eg, polycystic ovary syndrome [PCOS], thyroid disease, pituitary adenomas), coagulopathies, medications (oral contraceptives), trauma

What are common causes of abnormal genital tract bleeding during perimenopause?

Anovulation, polyps, leiomyomas, adenomyosis, cancer

What are common causes of abnormal genital tract bleeding in postmenopausal women?

Atrophy, polyps, cancer, endometrial hyperplasia, medications (hormone replacement therapy)

What are signs and symptoms of ovulation?

Thin vaginal discharge at mid-cycle and premenstrual symptoms, such as breast tenderness, bloating, and pelvic pain

What occurs to the endometrial lining during anovulatory bleeding?

Progesterone is produced by a corpus luteum after ovulation, and declining progesterone, in the absence of embryo implantation, contributes to cyclic menses. Without ovulation, estrogen, unopposed by progesterone, causes the endometrial lining to proliferate. Ultimately, the thickened endometrium outgrows its blood supply and undergoes partial shedding.

What is dysfunctional uterine bleeding?

Abnormal uterine bleeding in the absence of an anatomical lesion, systemic disease, or pregnancy; it is commonly secondary to anovulation

Which causes of AUB can be diagnosed using these tests?

    Pap smear

Cervical cancer

    Endometrial biopsy

Endometrial cancer or hyperplasia

    Pelvic ultrasound

Leiomyomas

    TSH and free T4

Hyperthyroidism and hypothyroidism

    Platelets, prothrombin time, and partial thromboplastin time

Coagulopathies

    Prolactin

Hyperprolactinemia, which can cause oligomenorrhea and galactorrhea

    Testosterone and dehydroepiandrosterone sulfate (DHEAS)

PCOS and ovarian or adrenal tumors

What are the medical options for treating menorrhagia in nonpregnant, hemodynamically stable women?

Treatment of the underlying disorder, estrogen-progestin contraceptives (with 30-35 mcg of ethinyl estradiol), levonorgestrel intrauterine device (reduces blood loss by 74%-97% after 1 year of use), NSAIDs (decrease prostaglandin synthesis leading to uterine vasoconstriction)

Your 19-year-old female patient is admitted to the hospital with a hemoglobin of 6.2 and menorrhagia. She has active uterine bleeding but is hemodynamically stable. What hormonal therapies can be used to reduce menstrual flow?

Combination oral contraceptive pills with 50 mcg of estradiol and 0.5 mg of norgestrel (or 1 mg of norethindrone) given every 4 hours until the bleeding decreases, then four times per day for 4 days, then three times per day for 3 days, then two times per day for 2 weeks; progestin-only pills (norethindrone acetate 5-10 mg or micronized progesterone 200 mg) can be given to patients in whom high dose estrogen is contraindicated; intravenous (IV) conjugated equine estrogen (25 mg IV every 4-6 hours until the bleeding stops but not exceeding six doses) is typically reserved for unstable patients.

ENDOMETRIAL CANCER

What are the risk factors for endometrial cancer?	Exposure to exogenous or endogenous unopposed estrogen (ie, without progestins), diabetes, hypertension
What are examples of exogenous estrogen?	Estrogen replacement therapy, tamoxifen
What are examples of endogenous estrogen?	Chronic anovulation secondary to PCOS, obesity, estrogen-secreting tumors
What are protective factors for the development of endometrial cancer?	Oral contraceptives (progestin suppresses endometrial proliferation), physical activity
What is the classic presentation of endometrial cancer?	A postmenopausal woman with uterine bleeding
What percentage of women with endometrial cancer present with AUB?	90%
What percentage of postmenopausal women with uterine bleeding will have endometrial cancer?	5%-20%
How do perimenopausal women with endometrial cancer present?	Abnormal uterine bleeding (eg, menometrorrhagia)
What are the diagnostic tests for endometrial cancer?	Endometrial biopsy (high sensitivity), hysteroscopy with dilation and curettage (the gold standard), transvaginal ultrasound
Postmenopausal women with an endometrial thickness less than 5 mm have a low risk of endometrial disease. True or false?	True

UTERINE LEIOMYOMAS

What are uterine leiomyomas (fibroids)?	Benign tumors composed of uterine smooth muscle cells

What are the three types of uterine leiomyomas?	1. Submucosal 2. Intramural 3. Subserosal
Why is the incidence of fibroids higher in reproductive age women than in menopausal women?	Estrogen and progesterone increase fibroid growth.
What are the risk factors for uterine leiomyomas?	Nulliparity (pregnancy promotes fibroid regression), obesity (increased estrogen exposure), African American race
How do OCPs affect uterine leiomyomas?	Combined OCPs reduce the relative risk of fibroids
What are the three typical signs and symptoms associated with uterine leiomyomas?	1. Menorrhagia 2. Pelvic pressure and pain 3. Decreased fertility
What bimanual examination findings suggest uterine leiomyomas?	Enlarged and irregular uterus
What imaging test can be used to confirm the diagnosis of uterine leiomyomas?	Transvaginal ultrasound (95% sensitivity)
Describe the medical treatments for uterine leiomyomas.	NSAIDs for pain control, GnRH agonists (eg, leuprorelin) to decrease bleeding and fibroid size, androgens (eg, danazol) to decrease bleeding
How do danazol and GnRH agonists work?	By decreasing pituitary gonadotropins
Will medicinal therapy improve fertility?	No
What are the surgical treatments for uterine leiomyomas?	Myomectomy or hysterectomy
Can a myomectomy improve fertility?	Yes
What is the name for the interventional radiology procedure for leiomyomas that injects small particles into the uterine arteries to decrease blood flow and cause regression?	Uterine artery embolization

POLYCYSTIC OVARY SYNDROME

What is the most common cause of infertility in women of reproductive age?	PCOS
What percentage of women of reproductive age have PCOS?	6%
What is the NIH criteria for diagnosis of PCOS?	1. Menstrual irregularity secondary to oligo- or anovulation 2. Hyperandrogenism (hirsutism, acne, male pattern baldness, elevated early morning testosterone) 3. Exclusion of other causes of hyperandrogenism, such as hyperprolactinemia or androgen secreting tumors
What other conditions are frequently associated with PCOS?	Obesity, glucose intolerance, endometrial carcinoma due to unopposed estrogen
What are treatments for PCOS?	Estrogen-progestin oral contraceptive pills can provide endometrial protection, contraception, and androgen suppression; weight loss can induce ovulation; metformin can address insulin resistance.

DYSMENORRHEA

What is dysmenorrhea?	Painful menstruation
What is the differential diagnosis of dysmenorrhea?	Primary dysmenorrhea, endometriosis, adenomyosis, uterine leiomyomas, chronic pelvic inflammatory disease

PRIMARY DYSMENORRHEA

What is primary dysmenorrhea?	Recurrent, lower abdominal pain occurring during menses without evidence of underlying pelvic pathology

When does primary dysmenorrhea typically begin?	Adolescence (with the prevalence decreasing with age)
What causes primary dysmenorrhea?	Frequent and prolonged uterine contractions from increased prostaglandins leading to myometrial ischemia
What are the clinical manifestations of primary dysmenorrhea?	Midline, suprapubic, crampy pain beginning before or with the onset of menses and lasting for 12-72 hours; only occurs with ovulatory cycles; can be associated with malaise, fatigue, and headache
What can be used to treat primary dysmenorrhea?	Heat to the lower abdomen, nonsteroidal anti-inflammatories (which inhibit prostaglandin synthesis), combination oral contraceptives

ENDOMETRIOSIS

What is endometriosis?	Endometrial glands and stroma implanted in areas outside the endometrial cavity
At what age does endometriosis typically present?	25-35 years
Why is endometriosis rare in premenarchal and postmenopausal females?	Ectopic implants are dependent on hormones
What is the most common site for endometriosis?	Ovaries
What are the next most common sites, in order of decreasing frequency?	Cul-de-sac, broad ligament, uterosacral ligament, fallopian tubes, sigmoid/appendix, round ligaments
What are the symptoms of endometriosis?	Three Ds: Dysmenorrhea Dyspareunia Dyschezia

What usually worsens the pain of endometriosis?

Menses (although the pain can occur at any point during the cycle)

Does endometriosis affect fertility?

Yes. Many patients are nulliparous.

What are the signs of endometriosis on physical examination?

Tender/enlarged adnexae, a retroverted uterus, tender nodules in the uterosacral ligaments and cul-de-sac

What is the gold standard for diagnosing endometriosis?

Direct visualization of the lesions during laparoscopy

How are endometriosis lesions described?

Raised, blue-colored mulberry spots or brown-colored powder burns

What are chocolate cysts?

Endometriomas formed when endometriosis invades the ovaries

Describe the fluid within chocolate cysts.

Thick, dark blood

What is the treatment for chocolate cysts?

Excision

Does a negative laparoscopy reliably exclude endometriosis?

Yes

Which medicines are used to treat endometriosis?

Combination oral contraceptive pills (OCPs)/progestin, androgens (danazol), GnRH agonists

What additional class of medications can provide symptomatic relief in endometriosis?

NSAIDs

How do danazol and GnRH agonists work?

Inhibit pituitary gonadotropin secretion leading to decreased ovarian estrogen production

Are danazol and GnRH agonists as equally effective as OCPs?

Yes. But they have more side effects.

What are side effects of danazol and GnRH agonists?

Hot flashes, vaginal atrophy, decreased bone density

When is it appropriate to refer the patient for surgery?

Failed medical management, severe pain, desired pregnancy

What is the conservative surgical option for patients who desire pregnancy?

Laparoscopic ablation and excision of implants and adhesions

What is the definitive surgical option?

Hysterectomy with or without salpingo-oophorectomy

CHAPTER 28

Family Planning

CONTRACEPTION

How does progesterone work as a contraceptive?	Suppresses LH to prevent ovulation, atrophies endometrium to prevent ovum implantation, thickens the cervical mucus to prevent sperm transport, inhibits peristalsis of fallopian tubes
How does estrogen work as a contraceptive?	Suppresses FSH to prevent emergence of a dominant follicle, provides stability to the endometrium to prevent breakthrough bleeding, potentiates the action of progesterone
How many weeks postpartum should a woman wait before resuming intercourse?	6 weeks
Which hormone should be avoided during exclusive breastfeeding because it decreases milk production?	Estrogen
What are birth control options for a breastfeeding woman?	Barrier methods, progesterone-only pill (POP), depomedroxyprogesterone (DMPA) injection, intrauterine device (IUD)
In a nonlactating woman, how early postpartum can you start an estrogen-containing contraceptive without increased risk of thrombosis?	3 weeks

If a woman using hormonal contraception prefers not to have her menses every month, what can you instruct her about timing of her pack/patch/ring?	Skip the 1 week of active pills or break from the patch or ring and immediately start the next pack/patch/ring
Do women have to take "breaks" from being on hormonal birth control?	No. Women who are healthy and do not smoke can use hormonal birth control continuously from menarche until menopause.

What percentage of sexually active women, using the following methods of birth control, will experience an unintended pregnancy in 1 year with typical use?

No birth control	85%
Male condoms only	15%
Period abstinence	25%
OCPs, patch, or contraceptive ring	8%
Depot-medroxyprogesterone acetate (DMPA) injections	3%
IUD	Less than 1% (ParaGard 0.8%, Mirena 0.1%)
Is male or female sterilization more effective?	Male, although the failure rate is low for both (male—0.15%, female—0.5%)
In which group of women is a cervical cap most effective?	Nulliparous women
Which lubricants are safe to use with latex condoms?	Water-based or silicone gels
Condoms are effective at preventing or reducing the transmission of which sexually transmitted infections?	HIV, gonorrhea, chlamydia, *Trichomonas*, syphilis, herpes, chancroid, HPV
Which birth control methods contain progesterone, but no estrogen?	Progesterone-only pills (micronor), DMPA injection, Mirena IUD, single-rod implantable device (implanon)
Which cancers have a proven associated decreased risk with combined oral contraceptive (COC) use?	Endometrial cancers, ovarian cancers, colorectal cancers

What other medical benefits do COCs offer?

Reduced risk of ectopic pregnancy and PID; treatment for acne, hirsutism, and androgen excess; reduced vasomotor symptoms in perimenopausal women; increased bone mineral density; decreased risk of hemorrhagic corpus luteum cysts; reduction in benign breast disease

What risks are associated with COCs?

Increased risk of cervical adenocarcinoma (rare) and hepatic adenoma; increased risk of venous thromboembolism; increased risk of myocardial infarction (MI) and stroke in smokers over 35 years old or patients with a history of HTN, diabetes, hyperlipidemia, obesity; severe migraines; reversible HTN; cholelithiasis

What class of COC may offer increased benefit to women with acne, hirsutism, or evidence of polycystic ovarian syndrome?

Drospirenone-containing pills (eg, yaz, yasmin)

Patients who have had a history of bariatric surgery should avoid what forms of contraception?

Oral pills—due to difficulties with malabsorption

What are contraindications to the use of COCs?

Smoker over the age of 35, uncontrolled HTN, migraine headaches with aura, SLE with antiphospholipid antibodies, hypercoagulable state, seizure disorder (on medication that induces hepatic enzymes), history of VTE, diabetes with complications, history of breast or endometrial cancer, prolonged immobilization, liver disease

What side effects might COC users experience?

Headaches, spotting, nausea, vomiting, breast tenderness, varicosities, VTE, stroke, MI, average weight gain is no more than in placebo users

How does DMPA affect menstruation?

Irregular menstruation during first several months and then possible amenorrhea, thereafter

What are some possible side effects of DMPA use?

Weight gain, acne, hirsutism, hair loss, mood changes, decreased bone mineral density

How often do DMPA injections need to be given for effective contraception?

Every 3 months

How often do the Ortho Evra patch and NuvaRing have to be changed?

Ortho Evra patch: once a week; NuvaRing: once a month

How does the ParaGard copper T (IUD) work?

Copper ions inhibit sperm motility and a sterile inflammatory reaction created in the endometrium kills the sperm.

For how long after insertion is the ParaGard copper T (IUD) effective?

12 years (approved for 10 years)

How does the Mirena IUD work?

Contains progesterone which thickens cervical mucus, alters endometrium, changes uterotubal fluid to impair sperm migration, and sometimes causes anovulation

For how long after insertion is the Mirena IUD effective?

At least 5 years

Who are candidates for an IUD?

Women in stable mutually monogamous relationships (low STI risk) who want reversible long-term contraception

What are side effects of an IUD?

Increased dysmenorrhea and blood loss (during first few months and more often with ParaGard), amenorrhea (after 1 year with Mirena)

A levonorgestrel-containing intrauterine contraceptive system (Mirena) can also be used in the treatment of what conditions?

Chronic pelvic pain, menorrhagia, endometriosis

The single-rod implantable contraceptive device containing etonogestrel (implanon) is effective for how many years?

3 years

It is a good contraceptive option for women with what conditions?

Hypertension, diabetes, VTE, cardiovascular disease, migraine headaches, sickle cell disease, HIV infection, seizure disorder

It can be beneficial for women with what conditions?

Dysmenorrhea

What contraceptive method can cause reversible bone mineral density loss?	DMPA
What contraceptive method has been shown to decrease sickling or painful crises in sickle cell disease?	DMPA
Approximately what percentage of pregnancies in the United States are unintended?	About 50%
What options are available for a woman who has just discovered she has an unintended pregnancy?	Continuation of pregnancy, adoption, elective abortion (some states require parental notification and/or consent for teens)
What is emergency contraception?	High-dose hormones given to prevent pregnancy after a contraceptive fails or after unprotected sex
What is the name of the only Food and Drug Administration (FDA)-approved emergency contraception pill being sold in the United States today?	Plan B
How does this work?	Stops ovulation, may prevent fertilization, may prevent implantation
Do the 0.75-mg pills need to be taken separately?	No. They can be taken one time in a dose of 1.5 mg.
What other hormonal options are there for emergency contraception?	0.1 mg ethinyl estradiol and 1.0 mg DL-norgestrel; two doses 12 hours apart starting within 72 hours of unprotected sexual intercourse
Who may purchase Plan B over-the-counter?	Men and women over the age of 18 years (women under 17 need a prescription)
How long after unprotected intercourse should plan B be taken?	Up to 120 hours, but it is more effective when taken as early as possible
How can nausea and vomiting be decreased when taking emergency contraception?	Take antiemetic 1 hour before the first dose.
What is the advantage of the progestin-only emergency contraceptive?	Decreased nausea, dizziness, and fatigue

What is the only contraindication to the oral combination method of emergency contraception?

Pregnancy

What is an alternative to hormonal methods for emergency contraception?

Insertion of the ParaGard IU up to 5 days after unprotected intercourse

How often after taking emergency contraception can a patient resume hormonal contraception?

Immediately after taking emergency contraception

INFERTILITY

What is infertility?

Failure to conceive after 1 year of unprotected sex

What percentage of couples experience infertility?

15%

What is the monthly probability of pregnancy among fertile couples?

20%

What is the cumulative probability of pregnancy among fertile couples after 12 months?

93%

What are common causes of a female etiology for infertility?

Anovulation or oligoovulation (polycystic ovarian syndrome, obesity); tubal interruption from PID, pelvic adhesions, or endometriosis; aging oocytes; uterine abnormalities, such as submucosal fibroid, septate uterus, endometrial polyp, or synechiae

How can you induce ovulation in an anovulatory patient?

Clomiphene citrate and gonadotropins

What is the mechanism of action of clomiphene citrate?

Blocks estrogen receptors and causes negative feedback on the hypothalamic-pituitary-ovarian axis to increase FSH secretion

What tests are indicated in the infertility workup for the following conditions?

Azoospermia

Semen analysis (semen volume, sperm concentration, motility, and morphology)

Anovulation

Midluteal serum progesterone level, urine LH surge detection, basal body temperature curve

Uterine abnormality

Hysterosalpingography, hysteroscopy, ultrasound

Tubal obstruction

Laparoscopy

CHAPTER 29

Dermatologic Complaints

ACNE AND ROSACEA

Acne is characterized by inflammation of what type of tissues?

Pilosebaceous units

Who gets acne?

Can affect all ages, but peaks in adolescence

What are the primary causes of acne?

1. Increased sebum production
2. Follicular hyperkeratinization leading to follicle obstruction
3. Growth of the bacteria *Propionibacterium acnes* in an anaerobic, lipid-rich environment
4. Inflammatory response

What are comedones?

Sebaceous follicles plugged with keratin and sebum

What does acne look like?

Open comedones (blackheads) or closed comedones (whiteheads), with papules, pustules, and cysts, with or without inflammation

What is the difference between open and closed comedones?

Open comedones are follicles with dilated openings from which sebum and keratin are easily expressed. They have a black appearance because melanin, in epithelial cells that were shed, is exposed to air and becomes oxidized. In contrast, closed comedones have microscopic openings so that materials are not easily expressed and melanin is not exposed to air, leading to skin colored papules.

What are some of the late manifestations of acne?

Scarring, postinflammatory hyperpigmentation

Is acne caused by chocolate and fatty foods?

No

Can stress cause acne exacerbations?

Yes, likely due to corticotropin-releasing hormone's effect on sebaceous glands

What medications can be associated with acne exacerbations?

Lithium, phenytoin, glucocorticoids, androgens

What is concerning about a patient with persistent acne and hirsutism?

An underlying diagnosis of hyperandrogenism should be considered. This presentation may be secondary to polycystic ovarian syndrome (PCOS) or androgen secreting tumors, including adrenal or ovarian tumors.

Where on the body does acne most commonly occur?

Areas with a high density of sebaceous glands: face, neck, upper arms, chest, back

What are initial topical regimens for acne?

Retinoid (adapalene, tazarotene, tretinoin) and benzoyl peroxide

What topical medications can be added for inflammatory acne?

Antibiotics (erythromycin or clindamycin). These should be used with topical retinoids (due to the increased efficacy of combination therapy) or topical benzoyl peroxide (to decrease the incidence of antibiotic resistance).

What can be used for more severe acne?

Oral antibiotics (minocycline, tetracycline, erythromycin, or doxycycline). To decrease antibiotic resistance, use for less than 6 months and add topical benzoyl peroxide.

What is isotretinoin?

A 13-cis retinoic acid that is a highly effective oral treatment for acne

What are the indications for isotretinoin therapy?

Recalcitrant acne (less than 50% improvement after 6 months of therapy with combined oral and topical antibiotics), scarring acne, acne with undue psychological distress, Gram-negative folliculitis

What are the FDA pregnancy risk categories for acne medications?

Class B: erythromycin, clindamycin

Class C: benzoyl peroxide

Class X: isotretinoin and tazarotene

What is the name for the chronic skin disease of the facial pilosebaceous units leading to flushing, telangiectasia, follicular papules, and in more severe cases, lymphedema and rhinophyma (enlarged nose)?

Acne rosacea

Who gets rosacea?

The age of onset is 30-50 years and is more common in females than males.

Are acne vulgaris and acne rosacea related?

No. But they can coexist. Rosacea has *no* comedones.

What triggers can exacerbate the vasodilatation associated with rosacea?

Hot/spicy foods, alcohol, temperature extremes, stress

What is the treatment for rosacea?

Avoiding triggers, topical and oral antibiotics (metronidazole, tetracycline, minocycline), isotretinoin for severe disease, surgery for rhinophyma

SUPERFICIAL FUNGAL INFECTIONS

How can superficial fungal infections be diagnosed in the office using microscopy?

Combine loose hair, scale, or subungual debris with 1-2 drops of 10%-20% KOH on a slide. Gently heat the slide and look for septate, branching, rod-shaped fungal elements (hyphae).

What is a dermatophyte?

A fungus capable of living on the keratin found in hair, skin, and nails

What three genera of fungi are collectively referred to as dermatophytes?

1. *Microsporum*
2. *Trichophyton*
3. *Epidermophyton*

Which dermatophyte is the most common cause of superficial fungal infections?

Trichophyton rubrum

Name the anatomic location associated with the following dermatophyte, or "tinea" infections?

Tinea capitis	Scalp
Tinea faciei	Face
Tinea barbae	Beard
Tinea corporis	Trunk and extremities
Tinea cruris	Groin
Tinea manuum	Hands
Tinea pedis	Feet
Tinea unguium	Nails

How does tinea corporis (ringworm) classically present?

Well-demarcated scaling plaque with a red, elevated, advancing border and an area of central clearing; may include pustules and vesicles at the margins

What is the most common cause of tinea capitis in the United States?

Trichophyton tonsurans infections

Describe the four classic clinical presentations of tinea capitis.

1. Seborrheic: scaly dandruff
2. Black-dot: patches of hair loss due to breakage at scalp surface
3. Kerion: tender, boggy scalp mass with enlarged posterior cervical lymph nodes
4. Favus: oval patches of hair loss with golden crust

What is the preferred treatment for tinea capitis?

Oral griseofulvin for at least 4 weeks

Describe the three clinical patterns of tinea pedis.

1. Interdigital: scaling in web spaces between toes
2. Moccasin-type: scaling on soles and lateral feet
3. Inflammatory/vesiculobullous: vesicles on lateral aspect of feet

What type of tinea infection is often associated with a dermatophytid reaction (id reaction = acute cutaneous reaction at distant site)?

Tinea pedis. It can result in a generalized immunologic reaction producing a vesicular eruption at distant sites (ie, hand dermatitis) that resolves with treatment of the primary infection.

How is tinea unguium treated?

Griseofulvin, Itraconazole, or Terbinafine

Excluding tinea capitis and tinea unguium, what is an appropriate treatment approach for most tinea infections?

Topical therapy with fungicidal allylamines (terbinafine or naftifine)

What are the potential complications of using combined steroid-antifungal agents?

Skin atrophy, steroid-induced acne, striae

What are the nondermatophyte organisms that typically cause tinea versicolor?

Pityrosporum orbiculare or *Malassezia furfur*

How does tinea versicolor present?

Hypopigmented or hyperpigmented erythematous macules with fine scale predominantly on the trunk

What is seen with a KOH preparation of tinea versicolor?

A "spaghetti and meatball" pattern with short hyphae and yeast

Describe the clinical patterns for these presentations of cutaneous candidiasis.

Candidal intertrigo

Well-demarcated confluent pustules on an erythematous base with satellite pustules at the periphery within skin folds

Thrush

Adherent, cottage cheese-like plaques on the oral mucosa

Perleche

Angular cheilitis with erythema, fissuring at the corner of the mouth

Paronychia

Infection of the proximal nail fold that presents with tenderness, erythema, and hyperkeratosis

What is the preferred topical therapy for superficial candidal infections?

Nystatin

What are the three most common causes of a red groin rash?

1. Tinea cruris (scale)
2. Candidal intertrigo (satellite pustules)
3. Erythrasma (*Corynebacterium* that fluoresces coralred on Wood lamp exam)

TOENAIL REMOVAL

What is an ingrown toenail?

A condition that arises when the lateral nail plate penetrates the lateral nail fold, entering the dermis

What are signs and symptoms of an ingrown toenail?

Pain, edema, exudates, granulation tissue

What are risk factors for ingrown toenails?

Improperly trimmed nails, hyperhidrosis, poorly fitting footwear, trauma (eg, stubbing a toe), subungual neoplasms, obesity

How should nails be trimmed to prevent ingrown toenails?

The nail should extend beyond the nail fold before the nail is trimmed horizontally.

How does hyperhidrosis contribute to ingrown toenails?

Sweat can soften nails resulting in the development of nail spicules, which can pierce the lateral skin.

How are mild ingrown toenails identified?

Patients have minimal pain, little erythema, and no purulent discharge.

What is an acceptable treatment for mild ingrown toenails?

Patients can attempt conservative therapy: soak the affected foot in warm, soapy water for 10-20 minutes daily and apply topical antibiotic ointment twice per day, or insert a cotton wisp or dental floss under the ingrown lateral nail edge

What is the treatment of moderate or severe ingrown toenails?

Lateral nail avulsion with or without matricectomy (recommended for recurrences)

What are the various ways to perform a matricectomy?

1. 80%-88% phenol (contraindicated in pregnancy)
2. Carbon dioxide laser ablation
3. Electrocautery

Should epinephrine be added to lidocaine to perform the digital nerve block?

No. Epinephrine causes vasoconstriction, and since digital arteries run in close proximity to digital nerves, there is a theoretical risk of causing digital ischemia.

What instrument is used to cut the nail?

Typically, nail splitters are used to cut from the distal nail straight back to the proximal nail fold.

What instrument is used to remove the lateral nail fragment?

Straight hemostats are used to grasp as much of the lateral nail plate as possible. Rotating the fragment toward the lateral nail fold while pulling straight out facilitates nail removal.

What are common complications of this procedure?

Postoperative patients with increasing pain, swelling, redness, or drainage should be treated for infection. Incomplete matricectomy can lead to regrowth of a nail spicule, which may need to be removed.

URTICARIA

How do urticarial lesions (hives) typically present?

Pruritic, raised, erythematous plaques with or without central pallor that can enlarge and coalesce

What is the hallmark of urticarial lesions as opposed to other red skin rashes?

Lesions disappear within a few hours after onset without leaving any residual marks

What is the time-course of acute urticaria and chronic urticaria?

Acute urticaria resolves within several hours without residual marks. Chronic urticaria comes and goes, but is present on most days and lasts for more than 6 weeks.

What are the two classes of antibiotics most frequently implicated in antibiotic-induced urticaria?

1. Beta-lactams
2. Sulfa-containing antibiotics (eg, bactrim)

Generalized urticaria following an insect sting should raise concern for what type of potentially life-threatening reaction with a future sting?

Anaphylaxis

How should you manage these patients?

Inform the patient about this risk, and ensure that they have epinephrine with them at all times.

What is the treatment of urticaria?

Remove the offending agent and use antihistamine H1-receptor blockers as first line, with H2-receptor blockers as adjunctive therapy; short-term course of systemic steroids can be used for patients who fail antihistamine therapy.

What are the characteristic features of urticarial vasculitis?

Painful rather than pruritic wheals that persist beyond 24 hours and leave a residual pigmentation

Name four systemic diseases in which urticaria can be a presenting sign.

1. Urticarial vasculitis
2. Systemic lupus erythematosus
3. Autoimmune thyroid disease
4. Cryoglobulinemia

How is angioedema different from urticaria?

Angioedema is deeper in the dermis and subcutaneous tissues resulting in more extensive swelling and edema

Describe four types of physical urticarias.

1. Immediate pressure—presents as dermatographism, often at sites of constricting undergarments
2. Delayed pressure—often affects the hands and feet
3. Cold—wheals in response to cold temperatures
4. Cholinergic—punctuate, pencil-eraser-sized wheals as cholinergic response to exercise, sweating , and/or hot showers

DERMATITIS AND ECZEMA

What is the clinical significance of the atopic triad of asthma, allergic rhinitis, and eczema?

The presence of one of these disorders is believed to result in a genetic predisposition to other atopic disorders either in the same patient or in the patient's family members.

In atopic dermatitis, a rash appears and subsequently becomes itchy. True or false?

False. Atopic dermatitis is the "itch that rashes." Symptoms appear before rash is present.

Describe the characteristic presentation of eczema in the following age groups.

Infants

Pruritic erythematous papules and vesicles that ooze and crust on the cheeks, forehead, and scalp (spares the diaper area)

Children

Lichenified scaly patches and plaques that ooze and crust on the wrists, ankles, buttocks/posterior thighs, and the antecubital and popliteal fossae

Adolescents

Scaling plaques on the face, neck, upper arms, back, and flexural creases

Adults

Scaling plaques on the hands, face, and neck

Describe some additional physical findings associated with atopic dermatitis.

Xerosis (dry skin), infraorbital skin folds (Dennie-Morgan lines), bluish discoloration of the periorbital skin, hyperlinear palm and sole creases, keratosis pilaris (follicular accentuation on the posterolateral arms and anterior thighs)

Name some common food allergens that have been associated with atopy.

Milk, egg whites, wheat, soy, peanuts

Name some common exacerbating factors of atopic dermatitis.

Excessive bathing, xerosis, environments with low humidity, emotional stress

What is the treatment approach for atopic dermatitis?

Eliminate exacerbating factors, treat noninflamed lesions with emollients, and reserve topical corticosteroids and topical calcineurin inhibitors for inflamed lesions

When considering treating atopic dermatitis with emollients, what is the optimal vehicle for the topical therapy?

Ointments (petroleum jelly) with zero water content followed by thick creams (eucerin, cetaphil) with low water content

Which areas of the body should not be treated with potent topical corticosteroids?

Thin skin of the face and skin folds can have irreversible skin atrophy with steroids.

A patient complains of red, papulopustules around the mouth and nasolabial folds that are mildly pruritic and sometimes painful. They have not improved with a trial of corticosteroids for contact dermatitis. What diagnosis do you suspect?	Perioral dermatitis
How should you treat this condition?	Stop topical steroids and start antibiotics (tetracycline, minocycline or doxycycline) for 2-6 weeks
Name the two types of contact dermatitis.	1. Irritant 2. Allergic
What type of hypersensitivity reaction is allergic contact dermatitis?	Type IV, T-cell mediated
Is allergic contact dermatitis always confined to the site of exposure?	No. It can be generalized.
What is the most common cause of allergic contact dermatitis in the United States?	Poison ivy
Which topical antibiotic is a common cause of contact dermatitis?	Neomycin-containing topical antibiotics
How is allergic contact urticaria diagnosed?	Prick test: a small amount of allergen is injected subcutaneously and is positive if a wheal develops within 15-20 minutes
Red, scaly plaques on the nasolabial folds, eyebrows, ears, or scalp suggest what diagnosis?	Seborrheic dermatitis
What is the treatment of this condition?	Shampoos with selenium sulfide or zinc pyrithione, or prescription shampoo with 2% ketoconazole for the scalp; topical steroid cream or lotion; tar shampoo; pimecrolimus 1% cream
In infants, this dermatosis is referred to as what condition?	Cradle cap

PSORIASIS

Describe the most common primary lesion of psoriasis.	Well-demarcated, pink plaques with silvery-white scales
Describe the primary components in the pathogenesis of psoriasis.	Hyperproliferation and abnormal differentiation in the epidermis with concomitant inflammatory cell infiltrates and vascular changes
What are the five different types of psoriasis and their characteristic signs?	Refer to the table below:

Plaque	Erythematous plaques with silver scale on scalp, extensor elbows, knees, and back
Guttate	Multiple, <1 cm psoriatic lesions on the trunk, classically after strep infection
Pustular	Sheets of superficial pustules and erosions, fever
Inverse	Lesions in the inguinal, perineal, axillary, and inframammary regions
Nail	Pitting in the nail plate

Approximately what percentage of patients with psoriasis also has psoriatic arthritis?	30%
Name three classes of drugs that can exacerbate existing psoriasis or result in psoriatic drug eruptions.	1. Beta-blockers 2. Antimalarials 3. Lithium
When evaluating a rash, involvement in which areas of the body should raise your suspicion for psoriasis?	The presence of lesions in the scalp, umbilicus, intergluteal cleft, and nail plate
What is Koebner phenomenon?	The development of psoriasis in areas exposed to physical trauma
What is the Auspitz sign?	Presence of bleeding within the psoriatic lesion upon removal of scales

Name some treatment options for mild, localized plaque psoriasis.	Emollients, topical corticosteroids, topical retinoids, calcipotriene, classical tar
What type of therapy should be considered in widespread psoriasis?	Phototherapy with ultraviolet light, oral retinoids, methotrexate, and immunomodulatory drugs (eg, etanercept, efalizumab)

HERPES ZOSTER

Herpes zoster, or shingles, is a reactivated form of what virus from the sensory ganglia?	Varicella-zoster virus
What does herpes zoster look like?	Grouped clear vesicles on an erythematous base in a dermatomal distribution
Where does herpes zoster most commonly occur?	The trunk
What are risk factors for herpes zoster?	History of varicella, age >50 years, immunocompromise
How does herpes zoster present in the prodromal, acute, and chronic stages?	Prodromal (2-3 weeks): stabbing/pricking pain in the involved dermatome Acute (3-7 days): new crops of lesions from papules → vesicles → pustules → crusts Chronic (months-years): post-herpetic neuralgia usually resolves within 12 months
What percentage of patients with herpes zoster will develop post-herpetic neuralgia (PHN)?	10%-15%. Incidence increases with age.
How can the diagnosis of herpes zoster be confirmed?	Tzanck smear, viral culture, or direct fluorescent antibody test
What is a Tzanck smear?	Scrape the base of a fresh blister and then spread on a glass slide stained with Giemsa or Wright stain to look for typical multinucleated giant cells

Can herpes zoster be spread?

You cannot give someone zoster, but you can transmit primary varicella from an active cutaneous lesion to a susceptible individual.

What is the treatment of herpes zoster?

Acyclovir initiated within 72 hours after acute vesiculation; pain control with analgesics, gabapentin, or tricyclic antidepressants

BACTERIAL SKIN INFECTIONS

What is cellulitis?

An acute infection of dermal and subcutaneous tissue characterized by red, warm, tender skin

What organisms most commonly cause cellulitis?

Staphylococcus aureus and *Streptococci pyogenes*

What part of the body is most commonly affected in cellulitis?

Lower legs

A young, otherwise healthy person presents with cellulitis of the arm. What should you suspect?

IV drug use

What should you think of in a patient with bilateral lower leg cellulitis?

Venous stasis dermatitis

What are the risk factors for cellulitis?

Disruption of the skin barrier, venous or lymphatic compromise, decreased immunity, a previous history of cellulitis

What is the treatment of cellulitis?

Initial empiric therapy with penicillinase-resistant semisynthetic penicillin or first-generation cephalosporin (vancomycin in severe infections or in areas with high incidence of methicillin-resistant *S. aureus*), surgical intervention with debridement for severe infections

What is the name for clusters of small, red, raised pustules and lesions less than 5 mm in diameter over hair follicles?

Folliculitis

What are the most common pathogens involved in this condition?

S. aureus, Pseudomonas (especially in hot tubs)

What is the treatment for this condition?

Warm compresses, topical mupirocin

What is the likely diagnosis when a patient has lesions that begin as papules and then progress to vesicles and pustules with honey colored crust?

Impetigo

When an abscess forms in the subcutaneous tissues below an infected hair follicle, what is this called?

Boil or furuncle

What is the most common pathogen involved in skin abscesses?

S. aureus

What is the treatment for skin abscesses?

Warm compresses, if small, incision and drainage, if large. Consider appropriate antibiotic coverage, if large or not resolving with compresses.

Intensely pruritic papules or burrows that commonly occur in finger web spaces, waist, and genitals should make you suspect what condition?

Scabies

What is the treatment of this condition?

Apply permethrin 5% cream over entire body from neck down and wash off after 8-12 hours, machine-wash clothing and bedding at 60°C.

HAIR LOSS

What is the most common cause of alopecia (hair loss)?

Androgenetic alopecia (male pattern baldness)

What are the approved treatment options for this condition?

Topical minoxidil (rogaine) and finasteride (propecia)

Can you use finasteride in women?

It is not approved by the FDA for hair loss in women. It is also pregnancy category X.

Diffuse hair loss of mature, terminal hairs is most commonly caused by what condition?	Telogen effluvium
What are some of the common risk factors for this condition?	Stress, weight loss, major illness, pregnancy, and traumatic events
Loss of 80%-90% of growing hairs is usually due to what cause?	Chemotherapy-induced alopecia (anagen effluvium)
What are common causes of traumatic alopecia?	Mechanical traction (hairstyles, braids), trichotillomania (self-induced hair pulling), excess use of chemicals or heat for styling hair
Smooth hair loss in discrete, round patches suggests what diagnosis?	Alopecia areata
This condition is associated with what other conditions?	Thyroiditis, vitiligo
What are common causes of permanent destruction of hair follicle (scarring alopecia)?	Bullous disease, discoid lupus erythematosus, folliculitis, lichen planopilaris
Hair loss in a discrete patch with underlying scaling of the skin suggests what diagnosis?	Tinea capitis

PIGMENTARY DISORDERS

Acquired skin depigmentation characterized by totally white macules that enlarge and can affect the entire skin is known as what disorder?	Vitiligo
What is the approach to management of this condition?	Protection of skin with sunscreen, cosmetic coverup to hide white macules, topical photochemotherapy with UVA, repigmentation with topical glucocorticoids or topical psoralens, photochemotherapy with PUVA for widespread lesions
What is the differential diagnosis of hypopigmentation?	Vitiligo, postinflammatory hypomelanosis, pityriasis (Tinea) versicolor, pityriasis alba, atopic dermatitis, psoriasis, cutaneous lupus erythematosus, seborrheic dermatitis, trauma, recent intralesional glucocorticoid injection

What is the most likely diagnosis of a hypopigmented macule with mild scaling that is often seen in persons with black or brown skin in temperate climates?	Pityriasis alba
A patient presents with hypopigmented macules and patches on their trunk for the last few weeks. They do not itch, but you notice a fine scale when looking closely at the area. What is the diagnosis and likely pathogen behind this?	Tinea versicolor
What is the treatment for this condition?	Topical antifungals
What is the name for well demarcated, hyperpigmented macules commonly found on the cheeks in women with pregnancy and the use of contraceptive hormones?	Melasma

WARTS

What virus is associated with cutaneous warts?	Benign epithelial hyperplasia caused by epidermal infection with human papillomavirus (HPV)
What is the characteristic appearance of a wart?	Flesh-colored, hyperkeratotic papule with vegetations, especially on the fingers and extremities
What is the pathognomonic finding for warts?	Black dots within the lesion, commonly referred to as "seeds," representing thrombosed capillary loops
Who is at higher risk for the development of cutaneous warts?	Individuals with decreased cell-mediated immunity, workers in specific occupations (eg, butchers, meat packers, and fish handlers)
How are warts transmitted?	A break within the stratum corneum allows penetration of the HPV virus through contact with humans or animals infected with HPV

How long does it take for cutaneous warts to resolve?	Two-thirds resolve on own within 2 years
What are the over-the-counter treatment options for cutaneous warts?	Duct tape, salicylic acid, cryotherapy, imiquimod, curettage and desiccation, electrosurgery, cantharidin, podophyllin, bleomycin, 5-fluorouracil

SKIN CANCER

In the evaluation of a suspicious lesion, what does the acronym "ABCDE" stand for?	Asymmetry Border irregularity Color variegation Diameter >6 mm Enlargement or elevation
What does the sun protection factor (SPF) indicate?	Measures the time a product protects the skin against burning. If you burn after ten minutes without protection, then wearing sunscreen of SPF 15 will theoretically allow you to stay in the sun 15 times longer before burning.
How should people protect their skin from the sun when outside?	Use sunscreen of SPF 15 or greater; wear hats, shirts, and pants when possible; avoid being outside between 10 AM and 4 PM.
How long before sun exposure should patients start applying chemical sunscreens?	30 minutes
What is the most common form of skin cancer?	Basal cell carcinoma (BCC)
What are the risk factors for BCC?	UV exposure, fair skin, individual susceptibility, previous radiotherapy, basal cell nevus syndrome, xeroderma pigmentosum, arsenic ingestion
What is the most common subtype of BCC?	Nodular-ulcerated (60%)
Where does it typically present?	On the face
What is the second most common subtype of BCC?	Superficial (30%)
Where does it typically present?	On the trunk

In what age group does the incidence of BCC peak?	60-70 year olds
What is the most common presentation of a BCC?	Shiny, pearly, or translucent nodule with telangiectasia
What are other skin findings that would make you concerned for BCC?	Sore that won't heal; red, itchy patch; elevated area with crusting; waxy area with tight, shiny skin
What are the treatment options for BCCs?	95% cured by simple excision or curettage and electrodesiccation. Recurrent lesions treated with Mohs micrographic surgery.
A scaly, crusted, "sandpaper-like" slightly elevated spot on sun-exposed skin that has appeared and disappeared and now reappeared in a 65-year-old male is most likely what lesion?	Actinic keratosis (AK)
What percentage of cases of actinic keratosis progress on to squamous cell carcinoma?	5%
What is the name and implications of an actinic keratosis on the lip?	Actinic cheilitis can develop into aggressive squamous cell cancer
What is the treatment of actinic keratosis?	Curettage, liquid nitrogen, topical 5-fluorouracil for 3-4 weeks, trichloracetic acid
An open sore that will not heal is most characteristic of what form of skin cancer?	Squamous cell carcinoma (SCC)
Both ultraviolet A (UVA) and ultraviolet B (UVB) radiation from sun exposure increase the risk of SCC. True or false?	True
Which type of ultraviolet light is emitted in tanning beds?	UVA
What are some of the risk factors for the development of SCC?	Chronic sun exposure; individual susceptibility; skin damage from burns, radiation, chronic irritation, or chemicals

What is the treatment of SCC?	Curettage and desiccation if less than 1 cm, excision with frozen section control, Mohs surgery, radiotherapy
What is the name of the SCC variant that consists of scaly, localized, slow-growing plaques associated with an increased risk of internal malignancy?	Bowen disease
What are the four types of melanoma?	1. Superficial spreading (70%) 2. Nodular 3. Acral lentiginous 4. Lentigo maligna
What type of melanoma is most likely to metastasize?	Nodular melanoma
What lesion presents as a rapidly enlarging vascular lesion following minor trauma, and is commonly confused with nodular melanoma?	Pyogenic granuloma
An African American male presents with a painless, dark brown discoloration under his toenail and on the sole of his foot. What is the most likely diagnosis?	Acral lentiginous melanoma
Where on the body are most melanomas located?	Trunk and legs
What is the major determinant of prognosis in melanoma?	Level of invasion (Clark level or Breslow thickness)
What is the treatment of melanoma?	Excision with sentinel node biopsy if more than 1 mm deep, chemotherapy if metastatic
What follow-up is needed after diagnosis of any type of skin cancer?	Check for development of new lesions every 3-6 months

RASHES AND EXANTHEMS

What is an exanthem?	The cutaneous manifestation of a systemic infectious disease
What are the six classic infectious agents that cause exanthems?	1. Measles 2. Rubella 3. Roseola 4. Varicella 5. Scarlet fever 6. Erythema infectiosum

Name the infectious agent of the following exanthems.

Erythema infectiosum (ie, fifth disease) — Parvovirus B19

Roseola — Human herpesvirus 6 (HHV6)

Scarlet fever — *S. pyogenes*

What is the first sign of measles? — Koplik spots—white papules on red base on the buccal surfaces

Describe the rash of measles. — Erythematous maculopapular rash that progresses cephalocaudally and then regresses cephalocaudally

What are the complications of measles? — Pneumonia, encephalitis, subacute sclerosing panencephalitis

Describe the rash of rubella. — Fleeting, discrete macules

When is rubella infection particularly dangerous? — Infection in pregnant women causes embryopathy in the fetus.

Describe the natural course of roseola. — High fever for 3 days followed by a rash that appears when the fever drops

What is the progression of the rash in roseola? — Starts on the trunk and spreads to the extremities

What is the treatment of roseola? — Supportive care

What is the classic rash of fifth disease? — "Slapped cheeks" and lacy rash (trunk → arms/legs)

What is the classic rash of varicella? — Crops of vesicles (dew drops on a red base) beginning on trunk

A patient presents with symmetric, violaceous macules on her eyelids. What is this rash and what condition should you suspect? — Heliotrope rash of dermatomyositis

CLOSURE OF SKIN WOUNDS

Prior to skin closure, what preventative measures should you take against tissue infection? — Wound irrigation, foreign body removal, and debridement of necrotic material

Are prophylactic antibiotics indicated for a clean, nonbite wound after suturing?

No. Antibiotics are used only if the wound is excessively contaminated, is in the mouth, caused by an animal or human bite, or the patient has vascular insufficiency or immunocompromise.

What are the different properties of suture material that you should consider when selecting one for wound closure?

Monofilamentous (Prolene or Ethilon) or multifilamentous (silk), tensile strength (higher number = thinner suture and less strength), memory (high memory = stiff, harder to tie, such as prolene), absorbable versus nonabsorbable

Describe the properties of the most common nonabsorbable sutures.

Refer to the table below:

Suture Material	Wound Strength	Knot Strength	Ease of Use	Tissue Reaction
Ethilon (Nylon)	Good	Good	Good	Mild
Prolene (Polypropylene)	Excellent	Poor	Fair	None
Silk	Fair	Excellent	Excellent	Significant

What theoretical advantage do monofilament sutures have over multifilament?

Multifilament sutures can facilitate bacteria between strands and increase infection rates.

What are examples of absorbable sutures (sutures that lose their tensile strength within 60 days)?

Vicryl, monocryl, dexon, PDS, maxon

What is the most common suturing technique for an uncomplicated wound?

Simple, interrupted sutures with nonabsorbable suture

After how many days should you remove sutures in the following locations.

Eyelids/Neck

3 days

Face

5 days

Scalp

7-10 days

Extremities

7-10 days

What are contraindications to the use of tissue adhesive for wound closure?

Complex laceration pattern, dirty wound, wound tension, wound length or depth >10 cm

What instructions should you give a patient after using tissue adhesive to close a wound?

Do not use antibiotic ointment over wound (leads to premature breakdown), return for wound check in 2 days, do not pull at adhesive as it starts to wear off

What is the wound closure method of choice for superficial skin flaps in the elderly?

Wound tape

What wound closure method is suggested for scalp lacerations and lacerations over hair-bearing areas?

Staples

Abnormal Test Results and Exams

CHAPTER 30

Abnormal Red Blood Cell Counts and Bleeding

What is anemia?	Reduced mass of circulating red blood cells (RBCs) demonstrated by decreased hemoglobin and hematocrit levels
What labs are included in the initial evaluation of anemia?	Complete blood count, RBC indices, and peripheral smear
What are the typical signs and symptoms of anemia?	Conjunctival and skin pallor, postural dizziness, fatigue, dyspnea (at rest or exertional), palpitations, tachycardia, high output congestive heart failure (CHF)
How can you determine whether or not the bone marrow is responding appropriately to anemia?	The reticulocyte index (RI) should be elevated.
What are reticulocytes?	Immature RBCs that normally account for 1%-2% of circulating RBCs
How do you calculate the RI?	Percent reticulocytes × (actual hematocrit/ideal hematocrit)
What does an RI <2% indicate?	Decreased RBC production (bone marrow is not responding)
What does an RI >2% indicate?	Increased RBC production: bone marrow is responding appropriately to RBC loss or destruction
What is mean corpuscular volume (MCV)?	The average volume of RBCs

What is the most common cause of normocytic (MCV = 80-100) anemia from decreased RBC production?	Anemia of chronic disease (ACD)
Describe the pathogenesis of ACD.	A chronic infectious, inflammatory, or neoplastic disease causes anemia by any one or a combination of the following: decreased response to or production of erythropoietin, bone marrow hypoactivity, shortened RBC life span
What is erythropoietin?	A glycoprotein hormone, primarily made by the kidney, which regulates red blood cell production
Besides ACD, what are other causes of normocytic anemia from decreased RBC production?	Bone marrow infiltration, aplastic anemia, chronic renal failure and other chronic disease, endocrine dysfunction (eg, hypopituitarism, hypothyroidism)
What is aplastic anemia?	Failure of bone marrow to make all blood cell types because the bone marrow stem cells are damaged. It can be idiopathic, genetic, or acquired.
What are the causes of normocytic anemia from increased RBC loss?	Acute blood loss, genetic and acquired hemolytic anemias, sequestration from hypersplenism

In hemolytic anemia, are the following typically increased or decreased?

Reticulocyte count	Increased
Lactate dehydrogenase	Increased
Unconjugated bilirubin	Increased
Haptoglobin	Decreased
Urine hemosiderin	Increased

Sickle cell disease, hereditary spherocytosis, hereditary elliptocytosis, glucose-6-phosphate dehydrogenase deficiency, and pyruvate kinase deficiency are all genetic causes of what type of anemia?	Hemolytic anemia
Paroxysmal nocturnal hemoglobinuria causes what type of hemolytic anemia?	Acquired hemolytic anemia

The following are examples of what
type of acquired hemolytic anemia
(autoimmune, alloimmune,
mechanical, drug-induced)?

Warm/cold agglutinin disease

Autoimmune hemolytic anemia

HELLP syndrome in preeclampsia

Mechanical

Blood transfusion with
incompatible blood type

Alloimmune

Penicillin, quinine, levodopa

Drug-induced

A Direct Coombs test for the presence
of antibodies against RBCs is positive
in what type of anemia?

Autoimmune hemolytic anemia

What diseases increase the risk of
developing autoimmune hemolytic
anemia?

Chronic lymphocytic leukemia, non-
Hodgkin lymphoma, mycoplasma
pneumonia, Epstein-Barr infection
(mononucleosis), cytomegalovirus
infection, hepatitis, HIV, autoimmune
diseases (eg, lupus)

What is microcytosis?

RBCs are too small (MCV <80)

What is sideroblastic anemia?

It is a genetic or acquired microcytic
anemia in which iron cannot be
correctly used to synthesize hemoglobin
and is characterized by the presence of
ringed sideroblasts (erythroblasts with
abnormal mitochondrial iron deposits)
in the bone marrow.

What is the most common cause of
acquired sideroblastic anemia?

Ethanol abuse

Overexposure to what heavy metal
commonly found in soil, batteries, and
cable covers can cause poisoning with
several toxic effects, including brain
damage (learning disabilities, seizures,
coma, death) and sideroblastic anemia?

Lead

What is the treatment of lead
poisoning?

Deferoxamine

What is basophilic stippling?

It is a classic peripheral smear finding seen in (but not unique to) lead poisoning. Accumulated ribosomal ribonucleic acid appears as spots on the periphery of RBCs.

What are the three main causes of microcytic anemia?

1. Iron deficiency anemia (IDA)
2. Anemia of chronic disease (normal or low MCV)
3. Thalassemia

Worldwide, what is the most common cause of IDA?

Parasitic infection

In the United States, what is the most common cause of anemia in children?

IDA from inadequate dietary iron

In the United States, what is the most common cause of IDA in adults?

Chronic blood loss

What is the most common cause of chronic blood loss leading to IDA in men and postmenopausal women?

Gastrointestinal (GI) bleeding

Besides a GI workup, what additional procedure is needed in the workup of IDA in a postmenopausal woman?

Endometrial biopsy

What is the most common cause of chronic blood loss leading to IDA in reproductive-age women?

Menometrorrhagia

What is the treatment for IDA?

Treat underlying cause of blood loss and give ferrous sulfate supplement

How long should you give a ferrous sulfate supplement in order to adequately replenish iron stores?

Continue treatment for 2 months after the hemoglobin corrects itself

In a person with IDA, effective iron supplementation should increase hemoglobin at what rate?

2-4 g/dL every 3 weeks

What is pica?

A craving for substances not fit as food (such as dirt, paper products, and ice), which is sometimes seen in IDA

What syndrome is associated with dysphagia and IDA?	Plummer-Vinson
What is the triad that characterizes Plummer-Vinson syndrome?	1. Esophageal webs (causing dysphagia) 2. IDA 3. Atrophic glossitis
Ferritin is an indicator of what mineral stores?	Iron
What is transferrin?	An iron-transporting protein
What organ produces transferrin?	Liver
What is TIBC?	An indirect measure of the amount of transferrin in the blood
How do you calculate percent TIBC saturation?	Serum iron divided by TIBC
What is a common iron panel profile for a patient with IDA?	Low ferritin (<40), high TIBC, low percent TIBC saturation (<20%)
What is a common iron panel profile for a patient with ACD (clue: iron is present but not available for use)?	Normal or high ferritin, low TIBC, normal or low percent TIBC saturation
What is thalassemia?	Anemia caused by reduced alpha (alpha-thalassemia) or beta (beta-thalassemia) globin protein production leading to decreased hemoglobin production
Thalassemia is more common amongst which ethnic groups?	Asian, Mediterranean, and African American
In a patient with thalassemia, what causes hepatosplenomegaly?	Extramedullary hematopoiesis
What lab test is used to diagnose thalassemia?	Hemoglobin electrophoresis
Why is it important *not* to use iron to treat a patient with thalassemia?	Patients with thalassemia already have a chronic state of iron overload

What causes the chronic state of iron overload in thalassemia?

Increased GI iron absorption secondary to accelerated iron turnover, multiple transfusions, or both

What is the treatment for thalassemia?

Transfusions and iron chelators

What is macrocytosis?

RBCs are too large (MCV >100)

What are the causes of macrocytosis?

Folate deficiency, vitamin B_{12} deficiency, drugs such as hydroxyurea and zidovudine (AZT), increased lipid deposition (liver disease, hypothyroidism, hyperlipidemia), alcohol abuse, myelodysplastic disorders

Folate and vitamin B_{12} deficiencies produce what kind of cells on a peripheral smear?

Megaloblasts (large immature RBCs) and/or hypersegmented neutrophils (at least five lobes)

Why does it take months for folate deficiency to develop?

Folate body stores (10,000 mcg) are small compared to the daily requirement (400 mcg).

What is the most common cause of folate deficiency?

Poor diet (classically associated with alcoholism)

What are other causes of folate deficiency?

Pregnancy/lactation (increased daily folate demand), drugs that interfere with folic acid metabolism (trimethoprim, methotrexate, phenytoin)

What is the treatment of folic acid deficiency?

Folic acid 1 mg PO daily for 1-4 months

Are neurological signs seen in folate or B_{12} deficiency, or both?

Vitamin B_{12} deficiency, since B_{12} is needed for myelin synthesis

What specific neurological signs and symptoms may be seen with B_{12} deficiency?

Loss of vibration and position sense, weakness, spasticity, ataxia, dementia

What causes the loss of vibration and position sense?

Degeneration of dorsal column tracts

What causes the weakness and spasticity?

Degeneration of corticospinal (upper motor neuron) tracts

Why does it take years for vitamin B$_{12}$ deficiency to develop?

B$_{12}$ body stores (5000 mcg) greatly outweigh the daily requirement (9 mcg).

What foods contain B$_{12}$?

Meat and dairy products

Where is B$_{12}$ absorbed?

Terminal ileum

What is the most common cause of vitamin B$_{12}$ deficiency in adults?

Pernicious anemia

What is pernicious anemia?

Impaired absorption of B$_{12}$ secondary to antibodies to gastric intrinsic factor (IF)

What are the other causes of vitamin B$_{12}$ deficiency?

Other causes of impaired absorption, such as gastrectomy or terminal ileal resection, competitive bacteria or parasites (tapeworm), and pancreatic insufficiency; poor dietary intake of B$_{12}$, such as in a strict vegan; impaired ability to use B$_{12}$

What are the treatment options for vitamin B$_{12}$ deficiency?

Vitamin B$_{12}$, 1 mg IM daily for 1 week—then 1 mg weekly for 4 weeks; vitamin B$_{12}$, 2 mg PO daily for 4 months; vitamin B$_{12}$ nasal spray (but comparative studies are lacking)

What is polycythemia?

Increased plasma concentration of red blood cells resulting in increased viscosity of blood (can eventually lead to thrombosis). Primary polycythemia (polycythemia vera) is a myeloproliferative disease.

What are the causes of secondary polycythemia?

Body senses relative hypoxia (high altitude, heart or lung disease, chronic smoking, etc), decreased plasma volume with subsequently increased relative red cell concentration (dehydration), erythropoietin or steroid secreting tumors, rare genetic causes

ABNORMAL WHITE BLOOD CELL COUNTS

What is leukocytosis?

Abnormally increased number of white blood cells

What are the causes of leukocytosis?

Leukemoid reaction (reaction of healthy bone marrow to extreme stress), reactive leukocytosis (as a response to fever, infection, etc), malignancy

Patients with infections can always have a high white count. True or false?

False. Many infections cause leukocytosis, but infections can present with low or normal white blood cells counts.

Allergies, asthma, and parasitic infections are associated with an increase in what type of white blood cells?

Eosinophils

Acute bacterial infections, especially pyogenic infections, are associated with an increase in what type of white blood cell?

Neutrophils

Viral infections are associated with an increase in what type of white blood cell?

Lymphocytes

Patients with leukemia can have a high, normal, or low white count. True or false?

True (depends on the subtype and stage of disease)

What signs and symptoms are common among people with leukemia or lymphoma?

Fever and night sweats, frequent infections, pancytopenia (fatigue from anemia, petechiae, easy bruising, etc), enlarged lymph nodes, hepatosplenomegaly, abdominal discomfort, loss of appetite, weight loss, bone pain, chest pain, shortness of breath

What white blood cell disease(s) are associated with the following?

Malignancy with translocation of Philadelphia Chromosome?

Chronic myelogenous leukemia

Tartrate resistant acid phosphatase (TRAP) positive and upregulation of annexin A1 (ANXA1)?

Hairy cell leukemia (when viewed under microscope, the malignant B lymphocytes appear to have tiny hair-like projections)

Bence-Jones protein, renal failure, hypercalcemia, anemia, lytic bone lesions, and pathologic fractures?

Multiple myeloma (malignant plasma cells)

Most common leukemia in the United States; more common in men and the elderly?

Chronic lymphocytic leukemia

Most common childhood cancer?

Leukemia (of which, acute lymphocytic leukemia is most common)

Reed-Sternberg cells, bi-modal age distribution of disease, Epstein-Barr virus infection?

Hodgkin lymphoma

Recessive disease (gene carried by 1 in 100 Americans), most common lysosomal storage disease, enzyme deficiency causes glucocerebroside accumulation in cells, hypersplenism with subsequent pancytopenia

Gaucher disease

The following are all examples of what type of hematologic malignancy: Waldenstrom macroglobulinemia, Burkitt lymphoma, Sezary syndrome, and follicular lymphoma?

Non-Hodgkin lymphoma

What is leukopenia?

Abnormally decreased numbers of white blood cells caused by decreased production or increased destruction of white blood cells. Leukopenia may be an isolated finding but often occurs with pancytopenia.

What is the most common subtype of leukopenia?

Neutropenia is the most common leukopenia.

What are the causes of leukopenia?   Refer to the table below:

Causes of Leukopenia

Cause of Neutropenia		Examples
Increased WBC destruction	Sepsis	
	Hypersplenism	
	Autoimmune disease	Systemic lupus erythematosus (antineutrophil antibody)
	Medications	
Bone marrow infiltration	Malignancy	Leukemia, metastasis
	Myelodysplastic syndrome	
	Myelofibrosis	
	Granulomatous infiltration	Tuberculosis, sarcoidosis
Bone marrow injury	Nonidiopathic aplastic anemia	Cancer chemotherapy, chloramphenicol, arsenic, benzene
	Radiation	
	PNH	
	Drug-induced neutropenia	
	Infection	HIV, mononucleosis
Other causes of decreased WBC production	Idiopathic aplastic anemia	
	Nutritional deficits	Folate, B_{12}

What is the mechanism of human immunodeficiency virus (HIV) transmission?

Contact with infected blood and body fluids, or vertical transmission from mother to fetus

What screening test is used for HIV?

HIV enzyme-linked immunosorbent assay (ELISA)

What confirmatory test is used for HIV?

Western blot

What groups of patients are at increased risk for HIV infection?

Men who have sex with men; persons who have unprotected sex with multiple partners, an HIV-infected partner, or a bisexual partner; persons who exchange money or drugs for sex; persons being treated for STDs; intravenous (IV) drug users; persons who received a blood transfusion between 1978 and 1985

Why is HIV-1 RNA viral load by polymerase chain reaction (PCR) a useful test in the following circumstances?

    Early HIV infection

ELISA and Western blot can be negative because antibodies have not been formed, but viral load is high.

    HIV in neonates

Cannot use serologic tests since mother's antibodies are passed through placenta and would result in false positive tests

What lab tests are used to monitor disease progression in HIV?

CD4 count, viral load

What determines whether a patient has AIDS?

HIV positive plus at least one of the following: CD4 count <200, opportunistic infection, B-cell malignancy, or Kaposi sarcoma

What is the most common opportunistic infection in HIV patients?

Pneumocystis pneumonia (PCP)

What is the best predictor of an HIV patient's susceptibility to infection?

CD4 count

What infections is a patient susceptible to when the CD4 count is

    Less than 500?

Candida, TB, herpes simplex virus (HSV), varicella-zoster virus (VZV)

    Less than 200?

PCP, *Toxoplasma*, *Cryptococcus*, *Histoplasma*, *Coccidioides*, *Bartonella*

    Less than 50-100?

Mycobacterium avium complex (MAC), cytomegalovirus (CMV), bacillary angiomatosis (disseminated *Bartonella*), CNS lymphoma, progressive multifocal leukoencephalopathy (PML)

What medications are given to HIV patients as prophylaxis for opportunistic infections, based on a CD4 count of

    Less than 200?

TMP/SMX DS daily (prophylaxis vs. PCP)

    Less than 150?

Itraconazole 200 mg daily (if in endemic area for histoplasmosis)

    Less than 100?

TMP/SMX DS daily (prophylaxis vs. toxoplasmosis)

    Less than 50?

Azithromycin 1250 mg every week (prophylaxis vs. MAC)

Name the four classes of medication used in HAART?

1. Protease inhibitors (PIs)
2. Nucleoside reverse-transcriptase inhibitors (NRTIs)
3. Non-nucleoside reverse transcriptase inhibitors (NNRTIs)
4. Fusion inhibitors (FIs)

Which vaccinations should be provided to all HIV patients?

Hepatitis A, hepatitis B, pneumococcus, influenza (intramuscular), tetanus

Which vaccinations should be avoided in HIV patients?

Vaccines which contain live viruses: measles, mumps, and rubella (MMR) and varicella (unless the patient is asymptomatic and with a CD4 count >200); nasal influenza vaccine

ABNORMAL PLATELET COUNTS AND ABNORMAL BLEEDING

What is the term for abnormally increased platelets?

Thrombocytosis (aka thrombocythemia)

What are the two main types of thrombocytosis?

1. Essential thrombocytosis (and other myeloproliferative disorders)
2. Secondary thrombocytosis (causes: iron deficiency anemia, hemolytic anemia, surgery, asplenia, "rebound" thrombocytosis following period of thrombocytopenia, acute or chronic infection or inflammation, cancer, drug reactions)

What are the major complications associated with essential thrombocytosis?

Numerous and dysfunctional platelets cause bleeding and thrombotic events.

Why do these complications not exist in secondary thrombocytosis?

Unless the cause of thrombocytosis (eg, cancer) in and of itself places the patient at risk for either bleeding or thrombotic events, the overabundance of platelets do not cause these complications because the platelets still function normally.

What is the term for abnormally decreased platelets?

Thrombocytopenia

What are the symptoms of thrombocytopenia?

Easy bleeding, which is most often noted at mucosal surfaces (nose bleeds, bleeding gums) and the skin (petechiae, purpura). Life-threatening hemorrhage may occur in severe cases.

What is the most common cause of thrombocytopenia in children?

Idiopathic (immune) thrombocytopenic purpura (ITP)

In ITP, what is the cause of platelet destruction?

Autoantibodies coat platelets and accelerate their clearance by macrophages that are usually found in the spleen and liver.

In ITP, is platelet destruction the only cause of thrombocytopenia?

No. There is also a decrease in platelet production.

What is the medical treatment of ITP?

Watchful waiting (some mild causes resolve spontaneously), or steroids and intravenous gamma globulin (IVIG)

What is the surgical treatment of ITP?

Splenectomy (the spleen produces autoantibodies and also removes platelets from circulation)

What two diseases are characterized by renal failure, thrombocytopenia, *nonimmune* (Coombs negative) hemolytic anemia, largely caused by blood clots within the capillaries and arterioles of many organs?

1. Thrombotic thrombocytopenic purpura
2. Hemolytic uremic syndrome

What are the mechanisms by which alcoholism can lead to thrombocytopenia?

1. Liver disease → splenomegaly → platelet sequestration
2. B_{12} and folate deficiency → decreased platelet production
3. Direct toxic effects of alcohol on platelets and bone marrow

What are the mechanisms by which cancer can lead to thrombocytopenia?

1. Primary or metastatic bone marrow lesions → decreased platelet production
2. Cancer treatment (chemotherapy, radiation) → destruction of bone marrow and blood stem cells
3. Complications of cancer such as disseminated intravascular coagulation

What are the mechanisms by which liver disease can lead to thrombocytopenia?

1. Portal hypertension → splenomegaly → platelet sequestration
2. Decreased production of thrombopoietin by liver cells → decreased production and differentiation of megakaryocytes

By what mechanism do nonsteroidal anti-inflammatory medications, such as aspirin and ibuprofen, reduce inflammation and fever but also increase the risk of bleeding?

Nonselective inhibition of cyclooxygenases (COX1 and COX2) blocks the pathways which produce prostaglandins and thromboxane. Prostaglandins mediate physiologic effects, such as inflammation and fever. Thromboxane increases platelet aggregation.

What is disseminated intravascular coagulation (DIC)?

A pathologic activation of the clotting cascade leads to formation of small clots throughout the vessels. Clots cause end-organ ischemia or infarction. Clots consume clotting proteins and platelets which causes abnormal bleeding.

What are the common lab findings of DIC?

Decreased platelets (consumption), increased PT and aPTT, positive D-dimers, decreased fibrinogen

What are the most common causes of DIC?

Sepsis, malignancy, trauma/surgery, obstetrical complications (eg, preeclampsia)

What is the most common bleeding disorder in the United States?

Von Willebrand disease

What is the Mendelian inheritance pattern of hemophilia?

X-linked recessive (thus, females are rarely affected)

What clotting factor is lacking in hemophilia A?

Factor VIII

Type B?

Factor IX

What are the major complications of hemophilia?

Severe internal bleeding (intracranial hemorrhage, hemarthrosis with significant joint damage), adverse reaction to clotting factor treatment, infection transmitted via blood transfusion (much less common nowadays)

CHAPTER 31

Abnormal Liver Function Tests

What are the most common causes of transaminase elevation?

Viral hepatitis, alcohol-induced liver damage, nonalcoholic steatohepatitis (NASH), hepatotoxic medications/herbs

Name some physical signs that may indicate that elevated transaminase elevations are due to *chronic* liver disease or cirrhosis.

Gynecomastia, testicular atrophy, spider nevi, asterixis, finger nail clubbing, ascites, organomegaly, palmar erythema

What liver function test is most specific for hepatocyte injury?

Alanine transaminase (ALT)

What causes of transaminase elevation result in an AST/ALT ratio >2?

Alcoholism and Wilson disease

What liver function tests are markers of cholestasis?

Alkaline phosphatase, gamma glutamyl transferase (GGT), and serum bilirubin

What tests are markers of liver function and protein synthesis?

Serum albumin and prothrombin time

The following lab results would suggest that a patient's elevated transaminases are due to what disease?

High ferritin, high serum iron, and low TIBC — Hemochromatosis

Low ceruloplasmin — Wilson Disease

Anti-tissue transglutaminase, anti-endomysium — Celiac sprue

High antinuclear antibody and anti-smooth muscle antibody — Autoimmune hepatitis

Low Alpha-1-antitrypsin — Alpha-1-antitrypsin deficiency

What patient characteristics and/or comorbid diseases would make you suspect NASH? — Obesity, hyperlipidemia (especially hypertriglyceridemia), diabetes mellitus

If a workup for elevated transaminases yields no specific cause and the patient profile does not fit a diagnosis of NASH, what is the next step in management? — Referral to gastroenterologist for liver biopsy

In the United States, what over-the-counter medication is the most common cause of drug-related acute liver failure? — Acetaminophen

For most adults, what is the maximum safe dose (g/day) of acetaminophen? — 4 g/day

What antibiotic is the most common drug cause of acute hepatitis? — Amoxicillin-clavulanic acid (Augmentin)

What medications (or classes of medications) used to treat diabetes may cause hepatotoxicity? — Acarbose, pioglitazone, sulfonylureas

What medications (or classes of medications) used to treat hyperlipidemia may cause hepatotoxicity? — Statins, nicotinic acid

Lab values showing an AST to ALT ratio greater than 2:1, hypoalbuminemia, markedly elevated GGT, elevated alkaline phosphatase, and macrocytic anemia are suggestive of what type of liver disease?	Alcoholic hepatitis
What vitamin supplements should be given to patients who consume alcohol regularly?	Folate and thiamine
What are the symptoms of hepatitis A?	Early signs: fever, malaise, headache, decreased appetite, nausea and vomiting, abdominal pain, diarrhea Later signs: jaundice, tender hepatosplenomegaly, pale stool
What is the mode of transmission of hepatitis A?	Fecal-oral (affected person may shed virus in stool for months, even when asymptomatic); food and water sources may be contaminated and produce epidemics
What is the incubation period of hepatitis A?	15-45 days
Children with hepatitis A are more often asymptomatic while adults are more often symptomatic. True or false?	True
It is possible for a hepatitis A infection to last several months; however, there is no chronic carrier state. True or false?	True
How can hepatitis A be prevented?	Meticulous hygiene, hepatitis A vaccine, hepatitis A immunoglobulin (only for travelers to endemic areas and for those with known close contact to an infected individual)
How is hepatitis B virus (HBV) transmitted?	Through infected blood (eg, drug use, tattoos, healthcare accidents), saliva, semen, and vaginal secretions (Note: while sexual transmission is common, perinatal exposure can infect infants.)

What is the incubation period of hepatitis B?	60-90 days
What percent of those infected with HBV will develop chronic liver disease?	10%
Chronic hepatitis B infection can lead to what complications?	Cirrhosis and hepatocellular carcinoma
Which virological marker is the first to emerge after infection with HBV?	Hepatitis B surface antigen (HBsAg)
Which virological marker correlates with the infectivity of HBV?	Hepatitis B e antigen (HBeAg)
Which virological marker allows you to distinguish between recent and chronic infection with HBV?	Hepatitis B core antibody (HBcAb)
Is HBcAb IgM positive in recent or chronic infection?	Recent infection
Is HBcAb IgG positive in recent or chronic infection?	Chronic infection
Interpret these Hepatitis B virological marker panels.	
HBsAg negative, anti-HBsAb positive, and anti-HBc IgG positive	Past HBV exposure
HBsAg negative and anti-HBsAb positive	Prior immunization
HBsAg positive, anti-HBsAb negative, and anti-HBc IgM positive	Acute hepatitis
HBsAg positive and anti-HBc IgG positive	Chronic hepatitis
How does an acute infection with HBV present?	Viral prodrome 4-12 weeks after infection; then with jaundice, scleral icterus, enlarged liver, and right upper quadrant pain
Which laboratory tests may appear elevated during acute infection with HBV?	Aspartate transaminase (AST), alanine transaminase (ALT), bilirubin, alkaline phosphatase, lymphocytes (especially atypical), prothrombin time (PT)

In the United States, what disease is the most common cause of liver transplant?	Chronic hepatitis C
What is the average incubation period of hepatitis C?	7-8 weeks
What is the mode of transmission of hepatitis C?	Most commonly through exposure of infected blood (IV drug use, blood transfusion, tattooing, organ transplant, etc) although exposure by other body fluids is possible
What percent of adults with acute hepatitis C develop chronic hepatitis C infection?	70% (even more develop persistent infection)
What is the initial test for diagnosis of hepatitis C?	Enzyme immunoassay (EIA) for anti-HCV
Why should patients with hepatitis C avoid alcohol?	Alcohol consumption increases the severity and rate of progression of liver disease. Alcohol also decreases the response to treatment (interferon therapy).
What complications may arise from chronic hepatitis C infection?	Cirrhosis and hepatocellular carcinoma
About what fraction of US patients have nonalcoholic steatohepatitis (NASH)?	Almost 1 in 4
Although NASH is usually asymptomatic, with what signs may it present?	Fatigue, malaise, right upper quadrant pain
What percentage of patients with NASH has hepatomegaly?	50%
How much do transaminase levels increase when a patient has NASH?	About 2-3 times normal levels (alkaline phosphates and GGT may also be elevated)
What is the preferred first-line and most cost-effective imaging modality for diagnosing NASH?	Right upper quadrant ultrasound (shows fatty infiltrates although does not determine severity of disease)
How is NASH managed?	Weight reduction, alcohol restriction, lipid and glucose control

CHAPTER 32

Abnormal Electrolytes

What is hyperkalemia?

Serum potassium concentration
>5 mEq/L

What factors place chronic kidney disease patients at risk for hyperkalemia?

They have reduced potassium excretion by the kidneys, are prone to metabolic acidosis, and are more likely to be on medications (RAS antagonists) that have hyperkalemia as a possible side effect.

What type of renal tubular acidosis causes hyperkalemia?

Type IV

In general, what are the causes of hyperkalemia?

1. Decreased potassium excretion: renal failure, renal hypoperfusion (heart failure, volume depletion), aldosterone deficiency or insensitivity, medications (ACEIs, potassium-sparing diuretics, NSAIDs)
2. Excessive release of intracellular potassium (acidosis, trauma, tumors, hemolysis, infection)

Hyperkalemia needs to be treated emergently when what factors are present?

Electrocardiogram changes (peaked T wave, loss of P wave, widened QRS), rapid rise in potassium, potassium >6 mEq/L, renal failure, moderate to severe acidosis

What medications are used to meet the following goals when treating *emergent* **hyperkalemia?**

> **Myocardial stabilization and prevention of fatal arrhythmia**

Intravenous (IV) calcium gluconate or calcium chloride (does not lower potassium)

> **Cellular uptake of potassium**

IV insulin (glucose is added to prevent hypoglycemia), IV sodium bicarbonate, nebulized beta-adrenergic (such as albuterol)

> **Elimination of potassium**

Furosemide or dialysis depending on the patient's renal function

What is the medical treatment of nonemergent hyperkalemia?

Sodium polystyrene sulfonate (PO or PR)

What is hypokalemia?

Serum potassium concentration <3.5 mEq/L

In a stable patient, oral potassium chloride powder (diluted in liquid) may be used to treat most cases of *hypokalemia.* **What is the approximate treatment dose for the following potassium levels?**

> **Less than 3.0 mEq/L**

20 mEq PO every 2 hours for four doses

> **3.0 to 3.5**

20 mEq PO every 2 hours for two doses

What are some common causes of hypokalemia?

Vomiting (bulimia, infection, hyperemesis gravidarum), diarrhea (infection, excessive laxative use), thiazide and loop diuretics, hyperaldosteronism, type I and II renal tubular acidosis

In the acute setting of hyperglycemia requiring intense insulin therapy, why is it necessary to administer potassium along with insulin?

Insulin promotes potassium uptake into the cells and decreases serum potassium.

Why does vomiting cause hypokalemia even though gastric fluid has little potassium?

Loss of hydrogen ions (acidic gastric fluid) → metabolic alkalosis → alkalosis causes potassium shift into cells

What are the symptoms of hypokalemia?

Weakness, fatigue, muscle cramps, constipation, arrhythmias (severe cases)

What is hypernatremia?

Serum sodium *concentration* >145 mEq/L. *Total* sodium may actually be normal or less than normal depending on the patient's volume status.

What is the difference between hypovolemia (aka volume depletion) and dehydration?

Hypovolemia refers to the loss of extracellular fluid volume (water plus sodium and other solutes) with resulting decreased tissue perfusion. Dehydration is a kind of hypovolemia but involves a disproportionately greater loss of free water to sodium, causing hypernatremia.

What are the common causes of *hypervolemic* hypernatremia?

- Hyperaldosteronism (eg, idiopathic adrenal hyperplasia, Conn syndrome)
- Excess sodium administration by physicians (eg, hypertonic intravenous fluid, parenteral nutrition, bicarbonate administered as $NaHCO_3$) or caregivers (eg, errors preparing infant formula)

What is diabetes insipidus (DI) and how does it cause hypernatremia?

Normally when the body senses dehydration, ADH (antidiuretic hormone) is released. The kidneys then concentrate the urine in order to retain more water. In DI, there is either no production of ADH (central ADH) or there is ADH insensitivity (nephrogenic DI). Inappropriately dilute urine is produced causing an elevation of serum sodium.

What is the major complication of treating hypernatremia too rapidly, especially if the patient has chronic hypernatremia?

Cerebral edema

What is hyponatremia?

Serum sodium *concentration* <135. *Total* sodium may actually be normal or higher than normal depending on the patient's volume status.

What is the mechanism of hyponatremia in patients with diabetic ketoacidosis (or hyperglycemia nonketotic coma)?

Even though glucose is not an electrolyte, it acts as a solute. So in a hyperglycemic state, serum osmolality is high. This draws fluid out of the intracellular compartment into the extracellular fluid. Serum sodium is diluted.

Describe the mechanism behind hypervolemic hypoosmolar hyponatremia.

In an edematous state (ie, CHF) there is a misperceived volume status. Total body water is increased, but *effective circulatory volume* is low. In response, the renin-angiotensin-aldosterone system activates (increases sodium and water retention) and ADH is released (increases water retention). Their net effect causes hyponatremia and further exacerbates volume overload.

What is the most common iatrogenic cause of hypovolemic hypoosmolar hyponatremia, especially in the elderly?

Thiazide diuretics

What is the major complication of treating hyponatremia too rapidly, especially if the patient has chronic hyponatremia?

Central pontine myelinolysis

When a patient develops the syndrome of inappropriate antidiuretic hormone (SIADH), do the following increase or decrease?

Serum sodium

Decreases

Serum osmolality

Decreases

Urine osmolality

Increases

What is pseudohyponatremia?

Elevated triglycerides or proteins → a decreased proportion of the serum is composed of water (and the sodium in it) → if the lab measures sodium concentration in whole serum (vs. serum water), sodium appears to be too low

What is the normal range for serum calcium concentration?

9-10.5 mg/dL

Lab values for calcium may be falsely low in patients with hypoalbuminemia (lab measures protein-bound calcium, not ionized [free] calcium). What is the formula for corrected total calcium in the setting of hypoalbuminemia?

Corrected total calcium (mg/dL) = total calcium (mg/dL) + 0.8 × (4−serum albumin [g/dL])

Does hypocalcemia occur with low or high magnesium levels?

Low

Does hypocalcemia occur with low or high phosphorus levels?	High
What is the most common symptom of hypocalcemia?	Neuromuscular instability (nerve and muscle twitching, muscle cramping, tingling)
What is Chvostek sign?	It is a sign of tetany seen in hypocalcemia. Tapping the facial nerve where it emerges just anterior to the ear causes spasm of the ipsilateral facial muscles.
What is the EKG hallmark of hypocalcemia?	Prolonged QTc interval
What are the two most common causes of *hypercalcemia*?	1. Hyperparathyroidism 2. Malignancy
What are the symptoms of hypercalemia?	Multisystem symptoms including "stones, bones, moans, abdominal groans, and psychic overtones": kidney stones, bone pain and osteoporosis, muscle weakness and fatigue, abdominal discomfort, mental dysfunction
In metabolic acidosis/alkalosis and respiratory acidosis/alkalosis, are hydrogen, bicarbonate, and carbon dioxide levels high or low?	Refer to the table below:

Acid-Base Disorder	H^+	HCO_3^-	CO_2
Metabolic acidosis	↑	↓	↓
Metabolic alkalosis	↓	↑	↑
Respiratory acidosis	↑	↓	↑
Respiratory alkalosis	↓	↑	↓

Of the above acid-base disturbances, for which is hyperventilation the compensatory mechanism?	Metabolic acidosis
Of the above acid-base disturbances, for which is hypoventilation the compensatory mechanism?	Metabolic alkalosis

How is anion gap calculated?

Difference between measured cations and measured anions:

$[Na] - [Cl] - [HCO_3] = $ anion gap

What is the typical acid-base disturbance(s) in the following scenarios?

    Diabetic ketoacidosis

Increased anion gap metabolic acidosis

    Opiate overdose

Respiratory acidosis

    Chronic renal failure

Increased anion gap metabolic acidosis

    Vomiting

Metabolic alkalosis

    Salicylate intoxication

Respiratory alkalosis and increased anion gap metabolic acidosis

    Lactic acidosis

Increased anion gap metabolic acidosis

    Pulmonary embolism

Respiratory alkalosis

    Chronic renal failure

Increased anion gap metabolic acidosis

    Neuromuscular disorder (ALS, multiple sclerosis, Guillain-Barré)

Respiratory acidosis

    Prolonged diarrhea

Normal anion gap metabolic acidosis

    Methanol, formaldehyde, or ethylene glycol intoxication

Increased anion gap metabolic acidosis

    Renal tubular acidosis

Normal anion gap metabolic acidosis

CHAPTER 33

Abnormal Urinalysis Results

What component of a urinalysis helps assess a patient's hydration status as well as the concentrating ability of the kidneys?	Urine specific gravity
When patients develop the following conditions, does their urine specific gravity increase or decrease from baseline?	
Dehydration	Increases
Diabetes insipidus	Decreases
Syndrome of inappropriate antidiuretic hormone	Increases
Urinary pH generally reflects the serum pH except in patients with what renal disease?	Renal tubular acidosis
What is hematuria?	The presence of red blood cells in the urine (according to the American Urological Association this equals three or more red blood cells per high-powered field in two out of three, clean catch, midstream urine samples)
When a dipstick test for hematuria is positive, why is it important to subsequently confirm hematuria microscopically?	Some conditions (myoglobinuria, hemoglobinuria) produce a false positive test for blood on dipstick. In true hematuria, microscopic analysis reveals intact erythrocytes in the urinary sediment.

Exercise-induced hematuria is a self-limited and benign condition that should resolve within how many hours?	48 to 72
In general, hematuria accompanied by proteinuria usually indicates that the blood loss is originating from the renal glomeruli. True or false?	True (glomerular hematuria often also presents with erythrocyte casts and dysmorphic RBCs)
What is the most common cause of glomerular hematuria?	IgA nephropathy (Berger disease)
In general, hematuria in the absence of proteinuria and RBC casts usually indicates a urologic or nonglomerular renal source of bleeding. True or false?	True
Give some examples of renal causes of bleeding that present this way.	Tumors, cysts, arteriovenous malformations, and infarctions of the kidney
When blood clots are present in urine, is the blood most likely glomerular or urologic in origin?	Urologic
What is the next step in management following a positive urine cytology test?	Referral for cystoscopy to rule out malignancy
Visualization of the upper urinary tract in a patient being evaluated for urologic bleeding is accomplished through what tests?	CT without contrast or intravenous (IV) pyelogram
What environmental exposures are associated with urologic malignancy?	Smoking, recreational, or work-related chemical exposure (eg, benzene)
A patient with hematuria and the following characteristics would make you suspect what disease?	
Family history of renal failure and cerebral aneurysms	Polycystic kidney disease
Family history of male renal failure and hearing loss	Alport syndrome
Fever, weight loss, rash, arthritis	Connective tissue disease (eg, lupus)
Severe flank pain radiating to the groin	Urethral distention most likely from stones
Palpable purpura of the skin, nausea, vomiting, diarrhea, blood in stool	Henoch-Schonlein purpura

What is the definition of proteinuria?

Abnormal urinary protein excretion (borderline proteinuria equals 150-300 mg/day, clinical proteinuria is >300 mg/day)

What is the difference between proteinuria and albuminuria and why is it important to make this distinction?

Proteinuria and albuminuria are abnormally high protein and albumin excretion in the urine, respectively. Albumin is a small protein and often the first to leak when there is kidney damage. However, not all patients with proteinuria have albuminuria (such as with light chain proteinuria [Bence-Jones]).

Urine dipsticks, which are often used in a clinical setting, offer a method to screen for proteinuria but may give false negative results under what conditions?

Dipstick analysis measures protein *concentration* so it can miss proteinuria if the urine is dilute. Also, the reagent on the test strips is highly specific for albumin and may miss nonalbumin proteins.

What are some causes of transient proteinuria?

Dehydration, exercise, emotional stress, fever, seizures, orthostatic proteinuria

What is the workup of asymptomatic transient proteinuria?

None, since it is rarely indicative of significant disease

What are the first follow-up tests in the workup of persistent proteinuria?

Spot urine protein to creatinine ratio (often preferred over 24-hour urinary protein excretion), microscopic examination of the urinary sediment, urinary protein electrophoresis (UPEP helps identify nonalbumin proteins), creatinine, and electrolytes

Nephrotic syndrome is indicative of glomerular disease. True or false?

True

What are the clinical signs that characterize nephrotic syndrome?

Proteinuria exceeding 3.5 g/day, hypoalbuminemia, edema, hypercholesterolemia

Light chain proteinuria (often nephrotic range) with or without renal failure presenting with the following signs and symptoms suggest the presence of what disease?

    Malignant plasma cells, renal failure, hypercalcemia, anemia, lytic bone lesions, and pathologic fractures — Multiple myeloma

    Restrictive cardiomyopathy, peripheral neuropathy, hepatomegaly, swelling of extremities — Amyloidosis

What is the most common cause of nephrotic syndrome in children? — Minimal change disease

    What is the treatment? — Steroids

Glucosuria (glucose in urine) occurs when the amount of glucose filtered by the glomerulus exceeds the ability of the proximal tubule to reabsorb it. Usually, this indicates that serum glucose is at least how high? — 200 mg/dL (very often an indication of uncontrolled diabetes mellitus)

What kind of cells in a urine specimen suggest contamination? — Epithelial cells

What is the most common cause of pyuria (>10 leukocytes/mL)? — Infection

What are some causes of pyuria not associated with infection? — Tumors, nephrolithiasis, trauma, glomerulonephritis, drugs (corticosteroids, cyclophosphamide), balanitis of noninfectious origin, urethritis of noninfectious origin

CHAPTER 34

Abnormal Pap Smear Results

What type of infection is the biggest risk factor for developing cervical dysplasia and cancer?	HPV infection with high-risk serotypes
What are some other factors that place a woman at high risk for developing cervical cancer?	Early intercourse, multiple sex partners, history of sexually transmitted infections, compromised immune system, early childbearing, oral contraceptive pills (OCP) use, smoking, intrauterine diethylstilbestrol (DES) exposure
Which HPV serotypes cause 70% of cases of cervical cancer?	16 and 18
Which HPV serotypes are considered "high-risk" for causing cervical cancer?	16, 18, 31, 33, 35, 39, 45, 51, 52, 56, 58, 59, 68, 69
The HPV serotypes 6 and 11 are not considered "high-risk" for the development of cervical dysplasia/cancer; however, are the cause of 90% of all genital warts (condyloma accuminata). Describe the physical appearance of these genital warts.	Single or multiple soft, fleshy lesions appearing in the anogenital area. Over time they may resolve, remain unchanged, or grow in size and number.
How can HPV warts be treated?	Imiquimod cream, podophyllin solution, liquid nitrogen, excision

Besides HPV infection, what factors place a patient at high risk for cervical cancer?

HIV infection or other immune suppression, history of intrauterine diethylstilbestrol (DES) exposure, history of treatment for CIN II/III or cervical cancer. Patients with these risk factors should have frequent cervical cancer screening.

All women who have undergone hysterectomy do not need Pap smears. True or false?

False. Only women who have had a hysterectomy with removal of the cervix for benign indications and who have no prior history of CIN II/III, or worse may discontinue routine Pap smears.

What is colposcopy?

A technique used to evaluate cervical dysplasia that involves a special microscope to visualize the cervix

What is the transformation zone?

The area between the old and new squamocolumnar junction, where squamous metaplasia commonly occurs

Why is it important to identify the transformation zone during a colposcopy procedure?

It is where most dysplastic lesions occur, and, therefore, a colposcopy is considered inadequate if the transformation zone is not visualized in its entirety.

Describe acetowhite lesions.

These are areas of epithelium that turn temporarily white when acetic acid is applied on the cervix. These areas are considered abnormal because acetic acid turns areas of high nuclear density white.

What are the visual differences between leukoplakia and acetowhite lesions?

Leukoplakia is also white but does not require acetic acid to be visualized. The lesions are also usually raised. Leukoplakia is a nonspecific finding but must be biopsied since it may be dysplasia or cancer.

Besides acetic acid, what other chemicals can be placed on the cervix during colposcopy for visualization of lesions?

Lugol or Schiller iodine solution (abnormal areas appear yellow)

What is the name given to abnormal capillaries that appear as fine or coarse dots often over acetowhite areas?

Punctations

A more severe abnormal vessel pattern which has a tiled appearance is called what?

Mosaicism

What procedures can be performed along with colposcopy?

Cervical biopsies and endometrial curettage

What is the significance of mucus-filled cysts on the cervix?

Nabothian cysts are a normal finding and do not require treatment

According to the American Society for Colposcopy and Cervical Pathology (ASCCP), what options are available for the management of atypical squamous cells of uncertain significance (ASC-US)?

HPV test is positive: colposcopy

HPV test is negative: repeat Pap in 12 months

HPV testing not done: repeat Pap in 6 months and 12 months and perform colposcopy if either Pap is abnormal

According to ASCCP, how does the management of ASC-US in adolescents differ?

ASC-US in this population should be followed up with annual cytologic testing. If the HPV testing was inadvertently performed, the results should not influence management.

Why?

The prevalence of transient HPV infection is high while the prevalence of invasive cancer is low in women 20 years of age or younger. Therefore, HPV reflex testing does not need to be performed in this population.

What is the initial management of low-grade squamous intraepithelial lesion (LGSIL) and high grade squamous intraepithelial lesion (HGSIL)?

Colposcopy

How is cervical dysplasia treated?

Laser ablation, cryotherapy, loop electrosurgical excision procedure (LEEP), cervical conization

CHAPTER 35

Positive Tuberculin Skin Test

What infectious agent causes tuberculosis (TB)?

Mycobacterium tuberculosis

How is TB transmitted?

Person to person through droplet nuclei (in general, extended close contact is required for transmission)

In general, someone with untreated active TB will infect 10-15 people a year. True or false?

True

If a patient does not have drug-resistant tuberculosis and is compliant with appropriate treatment, about how long after the initiation of antibiotics does the patient become noninfectious?

2 weeks

What organs does TB affect?

Most often, the lungs; however, it can attack any part of the body

What are typical symptoms of active TB lung infection?

Fatigue, weight loss, night sweats, fever, coughing, hemoptysis, chest pain

What is latent TB?

Infection with *M. tuberculosis* without active disease

10% of the world's population is infected with tuberculosis. True or false?

False (estimates are as high as 30%)

Even though patients with latent TB do not have symptoms, they are still contagious. True or false?

False. Latent TB is NOT contagious.

Why is it important to diagnose and treat latent TB?

5%-10% of people with latent TB can progress to active disease; active TB can be fatal. Treatment of people with latent TB is an important step toward the elimination of TB in the community.

How often should healthcare and medical lab workers be tested for TB?

Annually

Who else should be screened for latent TB?

People who have contact with a person known (or suspected) to have active TB, people with a compromised immune system (HIV infection, organ transplant, etc), recent immigrants from areas where active TB is common, people living in or who are exposed to people living in crowded conditions (homeless shelters, jails, etc), people with symptoms of active TB, intravenous (IV) drug users

What is QuantiFERON-TB Gold?

A highly specific whole blood test for TB that works by measuring a cell-mediated immune response in individuals infected with TB. It identifies both active and latent infection but cannot distinguish between the two.

What is the Mantoux tuberculin skin test (TST)?

An intradermal injection that screens for TB infection by inducing a delayed hypersensitivity reaction. Note: a screening blood test also exists, but it is less readily available and not the preferred method of screening.

How is a TST administered?

Tuberculin purified protein derivative (PPD) is injected into the volar surface of the forearm

How long after administration should a TST be read?

Between 48 and 72 hours

If a patient does not return within 72 hours after administration of a TST, what should be done to screen the patient for TB?

Reschedule another skin test as soon as possible (unless the patient had a severe reaction to the first test)

What constitutes a positive TST reading?

An area of induration (not just erythema) at the site of injection. For most patients, the area of induration must be at least 15 mm in diameter. For higher-risk patients (immune compromised patients, recent immigrants, drug users, etc), a smaller area of induration (ie, greater than 5 mm or 10 mm) indicates a positive result (specific tables are available from the CDC).

When should retesting occur for patients who have a known recent contact with a person with active TB but whose TST is negative?

12 weeks after contact (Note: in some cases, treatment for latent TB should start prior to the 12-week mark even if the TST is negative)

What is the BCG (bacille Calmette-Guérin) vaccine?

A TB vaccine used in some countries where active TB is common. Persons with previous BCG vaccination may have a false-positive TST; however, this should not preclude screening.

What is the next step following a positive TST result?

Determine if the patient has active TB by taking a history, examining the patient, and obtaining a chest radiograph

What is the preferred drug regimen (per the CDC) for treatment of latent TB?

Isoniazid (INH) for 9 months

What is the most severe adverse effect of INH?

Hepatotoxicity

What baseline laboratory tests are necessary before the initiation of INH therapy?

For most patients, NO baseline laboratory tests are necessary. Liver function (AST, ALT, and bilirubin) should be tested at baseline and then monitored routinely in patients with a history of liver disease (or who use alcohol regularly), HIV infection, or pregnancy (up to 3 months postpartum).

What is the purpose of monthly clinical monitoring of patients on INH?

To assess adherence to regimen, inquire about symptoms of peripheral neuropathy and/or hepatitis, and examine for signs of hepatitis

What are some symptoms of hepatitis?

Gastrointestinal upset (nausea and vomiting, abdominal pain), dark urine, jaundice

Patients on INH who are otherwise asymptomatic should discontinue INH if their transaminase levels reach what level?

Five times the upper limit of normal

Patients on INH who are symptomatic should discontinue INH if their transaminase levels reach what level?

Three times the upper limit of normal

Which medication can prevent INH-induced peripheral neuropathy?

Pyridoxine 25-50 mg PO once daily

CHAPTER 36

Cardiovascular Exam

CARDIOVASCULAR EXAMINATION

In order to obtain an accurate blood pressure (BP) reading, what percentage of a patient's arm circumference should be encircled by the BP cuff bladder?

80%

In the office setting, BP measurements are usually obtained while the patient is resting and seated upright. Describe the proper patient preparation as well as cuff and stethoscope positioning which is most likely to produce an accurate reading.

Patient has rested for at least 5 minutes. Legs are uncrossed and well-supported (not hanging from exam table). Clothing removed from upper arm where bladder cuff is placed. Arm is supported. Cuff is at the level of the heart. Patient is relaxed (not talking). Stethoscope bell placed over brachial artery in antecubital fossa.

When auscultating for Korotkoff sounds, why is it preferable to use the stethoscope bell (versus diaphragm)?

Korotkoff sounds are low-pitched

Which of the four heart valves is best heard at the following chest landmarks?

Left 5th or 6th intercostal space at the mid-clavicular line (apex of heart)

Mitral valve

2nd or 3rd intercostal space at the right upper sternal border

Aortic valve

4th or 5th intercostal space at left lower sternal border

Tricuspid valve

2nd or 3rd intercostal space at the left upper sternal border

Pulmonic valve

Name the diseases or abnormalities that first come to mind with the following physical examination findings.

Laterally and/or inferiorly displaced PMI	Enlarged left ventricle, most often caused by hypertension (HTN)
Pericardial friction rub	Pericarditis
Split S2 during inspiration	None (this is a physiologic split S2)
Split S2 during expiration (paradoxical split)	Left bundle branch block (most common cause), aortic stenosis
Wide split S2 (that varies with respiration)	Pulmonic stenosis, right bundle branch block, mitral regurgitation
Fixed wide split S2 (not varying with respiration)	Atrial septal defect (ASD) or right ventricular failure
Narrow splitting of S2 (increased P2)	Pulmonary HTN
Physiologic S3	Children, young adults, pregnant women
Nonphysiologic S3	CHF, enlarged ventricles, mitral or tricuspid regurgitation
Physiologic S4	Athletes
Nonphysiologic S4	HTN, coronary artery disease (CAD), aortic stenosis
Continuous machine-like murmur (congenital)	Patent ductus arteriosus
Mid-systolic click with late systolic murmur	Mitral valve prolapsed
Loud S1, opening snap, mid-diastolic rumble	Mitral valve stenosis
Bounding pulse, wide pulse pressure, soft but high-pitched early diastolic decrescendo murmur, best heard if patient leans forward	Aortic regurgitation
Harsh systolic murmur, increased with Valsalva, often with S3 and S4	Hypertrophic cardiomyopathy
Decreased pulse pressure, paradoxical split S2, harsh ejection murmur radiating to carotids	Aortic stenosis
Holosystolic blowing murmur at the apex radiating to the axilla	Mitral regurgitation

Holosystolic blowing murmur at the lower left sternal border radiating to the sternum; inspiration increases intensity	Tricuspid regurgitation
Diminished P2 with widely split S2 (or inaudible P2 and thus, no split), harsh mid-systolic murmur, most often found in children	Pulmonic stenosis
Harsh holosystolic murmur, very loud and often with thrill (congenital)	Ventral septal defect
HTN in the upper extremities with decreased pressure in the lower extremities, femoral pulse is slight or delayed, rib-notching on CXR	Coarctation of the aorta
Carotid bruit	Arteriosclerosis, arterial aneurysm, thyroid artery dilation, AV fistula

Describe the following findings of bacterial endocarditis.

Roth spots	Retinal hemorrhages with white centers seen by fundoscopy
Splinter hemorrhages	Narrow and straight lines of hemorrhage underneath the finger and toenail
Janeway lesions	Nontender, hemorrhagic macules, or nodules on the palms and soles
Osler nodes	Tender, red, raised lesions on the finger pads
What is pulsus paradoxus?	A patient's systolic BP falls more than 10 mm Hg (and causes weakening of the pulse) during inspiration.
What causes pulsus paradoxus?	Pericardial tamponade, asthma, shock, pulmonary embolism
What is Beck triad of cardiac tamponade?	1. Jugular venous distension (JVD) 2. Hypotension 3. Muffled/distant heart sounds

CHAPTER 37

Neurologic Exam

NEUROLOGIC EXAM

What are the components of a complete neurologic exam?	Mental status, cranial nerves, motor and sensory functions, reflexes
What information can be used to determine mental status?	Alertness, orientation, language, memory, abstraction, construction
What terms can be used to describe levels of consciousness?	Alert (normal level of consciousness), lethargy (arouses to your voice but appears drowsy), obtundation (arouses to gentle shaking), stupor (arouses after painful stimuli), coma (unarousable to painful stimuli)
Which type of aphasia is characterized by fluent speech but impaired comprehension?	Wernicke aphasia (also described as a word salad)
Which type of aphasia is characterized by nonfluent speech but intact comprehension?	Broca aphasia (also described as broken speech)

Name the function that corresponds to each cranial nerve.

Cranial nerve I	Olfaction
Cranial nerve II	Vision (assess visual fields and acuity and perform funduscopic exam), pupillary light reflex (mediated by cranial nerves II and III)
Cranial nerves III, IV, and VI	Eye movements
Cranial nerve V	Facial sensation and muscles of mastication
Cranial nerve VII	Muscles of facial expression
Cranial nerve VIII	Hearing
Cranial nerves IX and X	Palatal movement
Cranial nerve XI	Head rotation (sternocleidomastoid muscle) and shoulder elevation (trapezius muscle)
Cranial nerve XII	Tongue movement

What is the defect in internuclear ophthalmoplegia?

Lesion in the medial longitudinal fasciculus

What condition presents with internuclear ophthalmoplegia?

Multiple sclerosis

What symptoms will the patient with internuclear ophthalmoplegia report and what signs can be observed?

This is a disorder of conjugate lateral gaze in which the affected eye demonstrates impaired adduction. If the lesion affects the right eye, then the patient will report diplopia when looking to the left. On left lateral gaze, the right eye will not adduct. Convergence is generally preserved.

How can a central lesion of cranial nerve VII be distinguished from a peripheral lesion?

With peripheral lesions, the upper and lower muscles of facial expression are weak. With central lesions, only the lower muscles are weak, since the forehead gets input from the motor strips of both cerebral hemispheres.

What defect occurs following unilateral paralysis of the hypoglossal nerve (cranial nerve XII)?

The tongue deviates to the affected side (the tongue licks the side of the lesion)

According to the Medical Research Council scale, what strength rating should be given to a muscle with weak contraction that is able to overcome gravity but no additional resistance?

3 (0 = no contraction, 5 = normal strength able to overcome full resistance)

What signs are characteristic of upper motor neuron lesions?

Hyperreflexia, spasticity, weakness, positive Babinski (hallux dorsiflexes and the other toes fan out)

What signs are characteristic of lower motor neuron lesions?

Hyporeflexia, atrophy, fasciculations

Describe pronator drift.

Have the patient stretch out his/her arms with the elbows extended and palms facing up, and then close his/her eyes. Watch for 10 seconds for arm pronation or downward drift. A unilateral pronator drift suggests an ipsilateral upper motor neuron lesion.

How are normal reflexes graded?

2 (0 = absent, 4 = clonus)

Name the nerve root that provides sensation to these areas.

Thumb and index finger	C6
Middle finger	C7
Fourth and fifth fingers	C8
1st (great) toe	L5
5th toe and lateral foot	S1

What tests can be done to assess coordination?

Rapid alternating movements, finger-to-nose, tandem gait

Describe two rapid alternating movement tests.

1. With the patient seated, have the patient strike the palmar surface of his/her hand onto the ipsilateral thigh, raise the hand, turn it over, and then strike the back of the hand on the same place on the thigh. Have the patient do this movement as rapidly as possible.
2. Have the patient tap the distal joint of the thumb with the tip of the ipsilateral index finger as rapidly as possible.

Describe the finger-to-nose test.	Have the patient touch your index finger and then his/her nose alternately as rapidly and accurately as possible. Move your finger about so that the patient has to alter directions and extend his/her arm fully to reach it.
What is a tandem gait?	Walking in a straight line heel-to-toe
What physical exam findings suggest cerebellar dysfunction?	Dysdiadochokinesis (the inability to quickly follow one movement with its opposite), dysmetria (clumsy, unsteady, and inappropriately varying speed, force, and direction of movements during the finger-to-nose test), ataxic gait (one that lacks coordination)
The mini-mental state examination (MMSE) can be used to screen for which condition?	Cognitive impairment (or dementia)
How long does it take to administer the MMSE?	5-10 minutes
What is the maximum attainable score on the MMSE?	30

What are the MMSE questions pertaining to

Orientation?	What is the (year) (season) (date) (day) (month)? *[1 point for each; start with the year then narrow; maximum of 5 points]*
	Where are we (country) (state) (town) (hospital) (floor)? *[1 point for each; maximum of 5 points]*
Registration?	Repeat these three objects (eg, apple, car, chair). *Ask the patient to repeat all three after you have said them [1 point for each correct answer; maximum of 3 points]. Then, repeat them until he/she learns all three.*
Attention and calculation?	Start at 100 and subtract 7. Stop after 5 times. *[1 point for each correct answer; maximum of 5 points]*
Recall?	Repeat the names of the three objects. *[1 point for each; maximum of 3 points]*

Language?

Name these objects. *Point to a pencil and watch. [1 point for each; maximum of 2 points]*

Repeat the following: "No ifs, ands, or buts" *[1 point; maximum of 1 point]*

Follow this three-stage command: "Take a paper in your hand, fold it in half, and put it on the floor." *[1 point for each; maximum of 1 point]*

Silently read this sentence and do what is asked: "Close your eyes." *[1 point; maximum of 1 point]*

Write a sentence. *[1 point for a complete sentence; maximum of 1 point]*

Copy this design. *Show a picture of intersecting pentagons. [1 point; maximum of 1 point]*

INFANTILE REFLEXES

Describe the Moro reflex.

Sudden dropping of the infant's head in relationship to the trunk leads to abduction and extension of the arms and opening of the hands. This is followed by flexion of the extremities.

When does the Moro reflex typically disappear?

3-6 months of age

What is the palmar grasp reflex?

With the baby's arms semiflexed, place your index fingers into both of the baby's hands from the ulnar side and apply pressure into the palmar surfaces. The response is for the baby to flex his/her fingers to grasp your fingers.

When does the palmar grasp reflex typically disappear?

3 months of age

What is the rooting reflex?

With the baby's head in the midline, stroke the perioral skin at the corners of the baby's mouth and at the midline of the upper and lower lips. In response to a stroke at the corner of the mouth, the baby's mouth will open and head will turn to the stimulated side. When the upper lip is stimulated, the head will extend while the jaw will drop with stimulation of the lower lip.

When does the rooting reflex typically disappear?

4 months of age

What findings on physical exam suggest the presence of central nervous system disease in the infant?

Abnormal localized neurologic findings, late persistence of infantile reflexes, failure to elicit expected infantile reflexes, asymmetry of extremity movements, reemergence of vanished infantile reflexes, delays in reaching developmental milestones

SECTION IV

Individual and Community Wellness

CHAPTER 38

Statistics, Prevention, Well-Man and Well-Woman Exams

PREVENTIVE EXAM SCREENING

What is the United States Preventive Services Task Force (USPSTF)?

A panel that reviews literature and makes preventive care recommendations (for patients that are asymptomatic and generally at average risk for each disease)

In general, what factors influence USPSTF recommendations?

1. The degree of suffering from the disease (ie, death, disability)
2. The utility of the screening test (ie, sensitivity, specificity, simplicity, availability, cost)
3. The cost and clinical effectiveness of treatments for abnormal screening tests

How does the USPSTF grade its recommendations regarding which cancer screens should be routinely administered?

A = strongly recommends the service; *good evidence that benefit > harm*

B = recommends the service; *at least fair evidence that benefit > harm*

C = no recommendation for/against the service; *at least fair evidence that the service improves health outcomes but benefit ≅ harm*

D = recommends against routine administration of the service to asymptomatic patients; *at least fair evidence that harm > benefit*

I = insufficient evidence for/against routine administration

What are the recommended cancer screening protocols?

Refer to the table on next page:

Recommended Cancer Screening Per the USPSTF

Disease	Screen	Start Age	Stop Age	Interval (years)	USPSTF Grade	Comments
Colorectal cancer	Fecal occult blood test (FOBT) from three consecutive stool samples	50	75	1	A	The USPSTF recommends using one of these three modalities.
	FOBT + flexible sigmoidoscopy (FS)	50	75	FOBT: 3 FS: 5	A	
	Colonoscopy	50	75	10	A	
Cervical cancer	Pap smear[a]	21 (or 3 years after starting sexual activity—whichever is first)	65	At least every 3 years	A: sexually active with cervix D: total hysterectomy for benign disease	

Breast cancer	Screening mammography	50[b]	74[c]	2	B
	Clinical breast exam	40			I
	Teaching self-breast exam				D
Prostate cancer	Prostate specific antigen (PSA) and digital rectal exam (DRE)	50	75	1	I	PSA + DRE can detect early pathological changes but no studies have demonstrated ↓ mortality

[a]Pap smears obtain samples of squamous ectocervical (from the spatula) and columnar endocervical (from the cytobrush) epithelium. Dysplasia is most common at the transition zone between the ectocervical and endocervical epithelium.

[b]The decision to start screening before 50 should be an individual one, accounting for patient history and values (C recommendation).

[c]There is not enough data to assess the additional benefits of mammography in women ages 75 and older (I recommendation).

Who should be screened for abdominal aortic aneurysms (AAA) with abdominal ultrasonography (B recommendation)?

Males aged 65-75 who are current or former smokers (surgical repair of aneurysms ≥5.5 cm reduces deaths associated with AAA rupture)

Who should be screened for gonorrhea (B recommendation)?

All sexually active women (regardless of pregnancy status) who are at increased risk for gonorrhea infection (eg, age under 25 years, history of any prior sexually transmitted infection, new or multiple sexual partners, inconsistent condom use, sex work, drug use)

Who should be screened for chlamydia (A recommendation [nonpregnant], B recommendation [pregnant])?

All sexually active women aged 24 and younger, women aged 25 and older who are at increased risk

Who should be screened for HIV (A recommendation)?

All pregnant women, anyone requesting HIV testing, all adolescents and adults at increased risk for HIV infection. Men who have had sex with men, those who have unprotected sex with multiple partners, injection drug users, sex work, sexual partners with HIV, other STIs, blood transfusions between 1978 and 1985

Who should be screened for diabetes mellitus (B recommendation)?

Adults with sustained blood pressure (either treated or untreated) >135/80 mm Hg

Who should be screened for lipid disorders (A recommendation)?

Men aged 35 and older and women aged 45 and older with risk factors for coronary artery disease

Who should be screened for osteoporosis (B recommendation)?

Women aged 65 and older, women aged 60-64 with risk factors (such as body mass <70 kg, previous fracture, glucocorticoid use, smoking, excessive alcohol consumption)

What is the definition of at-risk alcohol drinking?

More than 14 drinks per week or more than 4 drinks per occasion for men, more than 7 drinks per week or more than 3 drinks per occasion for women

What questions can be used to screen for depression?

Over the past 2 weeks, have you felt down, depressed, or hopeless? Over the past 2 weeks, have you felt little interest or pleasure in doing things? Asking these two questions may be as effective as formal instruments.

Physician advice increases the rate of smoking cessation. True or false?

True

What treatments can be used to assist with tobacco cessation?

Nicotine replacement (patch, gum, inhaler, nasal spray), bupropion, varenicline

What medical conditions are contraindications to prescribing bupropion?

Seizures, anorexia nervosa, bulimia nervosa

What side effects are possible with varenicline?

Nausea is seen in 30% of patients (patients should take the medication after eating and with a full glass of water). Suicidality, depression, agitation, and worsening of preexisting psychiatric illness are rare but have warranted a black box warning. Check out www.uspreventiveservicestaskforce. org for more information about the USPSTF.

EPIDEMIOLOGY

What are primary prevention measures?

Measures aimed at preventing the development of a disease (eg, vaccines)

What are secondary prevention measures?

Measures aimed at detecting diseases early (eg, colonoscopies seek to detect early colon cancer)

What are tertiary prevention measures?

Measures aimed at reducing the negative impact of an already established disease and reducing disease-related complications (eg, monitoring for microalbuminuria seeks to identify and treat patients at risk for developing diabetic nephropathy)

Explain the following descriptive (hypothesis-forming) study designs.

Correlational

Uses population data, such as comparing a country's alcohol intake to its prevalence of coronary artery disease

Case report

Descriptive study of factors that could be related to an outcome

Cross-sectional

Assesses the outcome and exposure simultaneously

Can cross-sectional studies prove causality?

No, because the temporal relationship between the variables is unknown.

Give examples of the following analytic (hypothesis-testing) study designs.

Observational

Cohort and case-control studies

Interventional

Randomized controlled trials (RCTs)

How are patients in a case-control study grouped and evaluated?

Persons with a known outcome (such as cancer) are identified as "cases" and those without the outcome as "controls." The study compares the groups, looking for multiple potential exposures of the outcome.

How are patients in a cohort study grouped and evaluated?

Participants are divided into groups based on some common exposure (such as low vs. high fat diets). The study compares multiple potential outcomes of the exposure.

What are prospective studies?

At the study initiation, the disease has not occurred, and the study group is followed forward in time.

What are retrospective studies?

At the study initiation, the disease has occurred, and the researcher looks back in time to identify potential etiologies.

What is the term used to describe the following?

The percent of the population with a disease at a given point in time (# persons with the disease/# persons in the total population)	Prevalence
The percent of the population who develop a disease over a period of time (# persons who develop the disease/# persons who are initially disease-free in a population)	Incidence

DISEASE AND EXPOSURE

	Disease +	Disease −	
Exposure +	a	B	a + b = total exposed
Exposure −	c	D	c + d = total unexposed
	a + c = total with disease	b + d = total without disease	total

What is relative risk?	The incidence of disease in those exposed to a particular factor compared to the incidence of disease in the unexposed
How do you calculate relative risk?	Relative risk = $(a/[a + b])/(c/[c + d])$
When is relative risk used?	In cohort studies and RCTs
How do you calculate absolute risk?	Absolute risk = $(a/[a + b]) − (c/[c + d])$
How do you calculate number needed to treat (in cases where the exposure is a treatment or intervention)?	Number needed to treat = $1/$absolute risk
How do you calculate an odds ratio?	Odds ratio = $(a \times d)/(b \times c)$
When is an odds ratio used?	In case-control studies
Why are odds ratios used in case-control studies?	In case-control studies you cannot calculate disease development, so you cannot calculate relative risk. Odds ratios approximate the relative risk.

TRUE POSITIVE, TRUE NEGATIVE, FALSE POSITIVE, AND FALSE NEGATIVE

	Disease +	Disease −	
Test +	a = true positive (TP)	b = false positive (FP)	a + b = total with + tests
Test −	c = false negative (FN)	d = true negative (TN)	c + d = total with − tests
	a + c = total with disease	b + d = total without disease	total

What does a "false negative" result mean?

A person with a disease who tests negative for that disease

What does a "false positive" result mean?

A person without a disease tests positive for that disease

Define sensitivity.

Percent of those with the disease that test positive

How do you calculate sensitivity?

TP/(TP + FN) = TP/(everyone with the disease); see above table

Define specificity.

Percent of those without the disease that test negative

How do you calculate specificity?

TN/(TN + FP) = TN/(everyone without the disease)

What is more desirable in a screening test, high sensitivity or high specificity?

High sensitivity (*SnNOut*: in a sensitive [*Sn*] test, a negative result [*N*] helps to rule out [*Out*] disease)

What is more desirable in a confirmatory test, high sensitivity or high specificity?

High specificity (*SpPIn*: in a specific [*Sp*] test, a positive result [*P*] helps to rule in [*In*] disease)

What is positive predictive value (PPV)?

Percent of those with positive tests that actually have the disease

How do you calculate PPV?

PPV = TP/(TP + FP) = TP/(all those with positive tests)

What is negative predictive value (NPV)?

Percent of those with negative tests that actually do not have the disease

How do you calculate NPV?	NPV = TN/(TN + FN) = TN/(all those with negative tests)
How does disease prevalence affect PPV and NPV?	Increasing prevalence leads to increasing PPV, decreasing prevalence leads to increasing NPV
What are POEMs?	Patient Oriented Evidence that Matters. This is a method for identifying articles that are particularly high-yield for primary care physicians.
How are POEMs identified?	A POEM will meet the following criteria and warrants a closer look:

1. Would your patient care about the study's outcome (ie, death rather than plaque thickness)?
2. Is it something you see in your practice at least once every 6 months?
3. If true, would the study's findings change what you do (or are you already doing what the study is telling you to do)?

VACCINES IN ADULTS AND CHILDREN

What are examples of live vaccines?	Measles, mumps, and rubella (MMR); sabin oral polio vaccine; varicella vaccine; rotavirus
Why is the oral polio vaccine no longer distributed in the United States?	Increased risk of vaccine-associated paralytic poliomyelitis
Which populations should avoid live vaccines?	Pregnant women, the immunocompromised, and the close contacts of the immunocompromised
What are the standard childhood immunizations?	MMR; varicella; hepatitis B; hepatitis A; *Haemophilus influenzae* type b (Hib); inactivated polio (IPV); pneumococcal conjugate vaccine (PCV7); diphtheria, tetanus, and acellular pertussis (DTaP); rotavirus; influenza

What is the dosing schedule for the MMR vaccine?	Two doses: 12-15 months old and 4-6 years old
What is the dosing schedule for the varicella vaccine?	Two doses: 12-15 months old and 4-6 years old
Live vaccines are contraindicated in patients with HIV. True or false?	False. MMR and the varicella vaccine can be given to HIV patients with CD4 T-cell counts >200 cells/mL.
What is the dosing schedule for the oral pentavalent rotavirus vaccine?	Three doses: 2, 4, and 6 months old. The series should not be started after the age of 12 weeks, and the final dose should be given by the age of 32 weeks.
What is the dosing schedule for the hepatitis B vaccine?	Three doses: 0-1 month old, 1-4 months old, and 6-18 months old
What is the management of a child born to an HBsAg positive mom?	Give the first dose of the hepatitis B vaccine and hepatitis B immunoglobulin (HBIG) at birth
What is the dosing schedule for the hepatitis A vaccine?	Two doses: 1 year old and then 6-18 months later
What is the dosing schedule for DTaP?	Five doses: 2, 4, 6, 15-18 months old, and 4-6 years old; give Td (tetanus and diphtheria toxoids) boosters at age 11-12 years and then every 10 years
What is the dosing schedule for the Hib vaccine?	Four doses: 2, 4, 6, and 12-15 months old
Since the introduction of the Hib vaccine in 1987, the number of Hib (a cause of meningitis and epiglottitis) cases in children less than 5 years old has decreased by what percentage?	99%
What is the dosing schedule for the IPV?	Four doses: 2, 4, and 6 months old; 4-6 years old
What is the dosing schedule for PCV7?	Four doses: 2, 4, 6, and 12-15 months old

Who should be offered the conjugated quadrivalent meningococcal polysaccharide vaccine (MCV4)?

11-12 year olds, at age 13-18 if not previously vaccinated, previously unvaccinated college freshmen living in dorms, to children aged 2-10 with persistent complement component deficiency or anatomic or functional asplenia

Who should be offered revaccination with MCV4?

If the first dose was administered at age 2-6, then revaccinate children who remain at risk after 3 years. If the first dose was administered at age 7 years or older, then revaccinate after 5 years. Patients who remain at increased risk for meningococcal disease should be revaccinated at 5-year intervals.

Asplenic patients are particularly vulnerable to what kind of infections?

Encapsulated bacterial infections

What is the dosing schedule for the influenza vaccine?

Everyone 6 months of age and older should get an influenza vaccine every year (influenza has a high rate of mutation).

What time of year should the influenza vaccine be administered?

Once it is available for a particular year, the vaccine may be administered at anytime (the earlier the better) before or during the influenza season, which usually peaks in the fall/winter months.

Which patients should not be offered the influenza vaccine?

Patients with anaphylaxis to eggs (since the vaccine is prepared from viruses grown in eggs)

Who should be offered the H1N1 influenza vaccine?

All patients 6 months of age and older

What is the current recommendation for HPV vaccination?

HPV2 (protects against types 16 and 18) or HPV4 (protects against types 6, 11, 16, and 18) is recommended for females at age 11 or 12 years old; however, catch up vaccination can be done up until age 26.

When should the second and third doses of HPV vaccine be administered?

Second dose 2 months after the first and the third dose 6 months after the first

Can the HPV vaccine be administered to males?

HPV4 may be administered to males (9-26 years old) to help prevent genital warts

Can females over the age of 26 receive the "quadrivalent" vaccine?

Yes; however, studies are still ongoing proving safety of efficacy in this age group

Should the vaccine be administered to those who have a history of genital warts, abnormal Pap, and/or positive HPV DNA test?

Yes. Vaccination is less effective for those who have already been infected with one or more of the HPV types; however, the vaccine should still be administered since there is still some protection conferred against the other HPV types.

Why should females who have received the quadrivalent vaccine still be screened for cervical cancer?

The vaccine does not protect against all HPV types that cause cancer. Patients may not have received all the doses of the vaccine. Patients who already have acquired HPV may not get the vaccine's full benefit.

Which patients should be offered pneumococcal polysaccharide vaccine (PPV23)?

Adults ≥65 years old; patients with chronic respiratory disease (including asthma), alcoholism, cardiovascular disease, diabetes, chronic liver disease, chronic renal failure, cochlear implants, and nephrotic syndrome; nursing home residents; immunocompromised patients; asplenic patients; patients who smoke cigarettes

What are the indications for revaccination with PPV23?

Patient received the vaccine ≥5 years previously and was < 65 years old at the time of vaccination, immunocompromised, asplenia, postorgan or bone marrow transplantation

Why can you not use PPV23 in children?

PPV23 contains polysaccharide antigens that are not immunogenic in children <2 years old (PCV7 contains 7 capsular polysaccharides conjugated to a protein)

Which patients should be offered a single dose of the zoster vaccine to prevent shingles and postherpetic neuralgia?

Adults aged 60 years and older

Which patients should not receive the shingles vaccine?

Pregnant women, those with a history of anaphylaxis to gelatin or neomycin, immunodeficient patient (including those with AIDS and on immunosuppressive therapies)

The shingles vaccine can be given to those with a history of shingles. True or false?

True. The Advisory Committee on Immunization Practices recommends offering the vaccine regardless of prior shingles history though use of the vaccine has not specifically been studied in this population.

Check out www.cdc.gov/vaccines for more information about vaccines.

INFECTIVE ENDOCARDITIS (IE) PROPHYLAXIS

What is the theoretical basis for IE prophylaxis?

Transient bacteremia (especially *Streptococcus viridans*) is common after invasive procedures.

According to the American Heart Association (AHA), patients with what conditions are at the highest risk for IE?

Prosthetic heart valves, prior history of IE, unrepaired cyanotic congenital heart disease, completely repaired congenital heart defects with prosthetic material (during the first 6 months after the procedure), repaired congenital heart disease with residual defects, cardiac transplantation recipients who develop cardiac valvulopathy

Which patients should receive prophylaxis?

Only patients at the highest risk undergoing high-risk procedures

Following the 2007 AHA guidelines, which common valvular lesions no longer require antimicrobial prophylaxis?

Bicuspid aortic valve, aortic/mitral valve disease

What high-risk procedures are most likely to result in transient bacteremia?

All dental procedures involving manipulation of either gingival tissue or the periapical region of teeth or perforation of the oral mucosa, procedures of the respiratory tract involving incision of the respiratory mucosas, procedures in patients with ongoing gastrointestinal (GI) or genitourinary (GU) infections, procedures on infected skin or musculoskeletal tissue, surgery to place prosthetic heart valves or prosthetic intravascular or intracardiac materials

What is the recommended IE prophylaxis for dental procedures in patients at the highest risk?

Amoxicillin 2 g, 1 hour prior to the procedure

Check out www.americanheart.org/presenter.jhtml?identifier=4436 for more information from the American Heart Association about endocarditis prophylaxis.

CHAPTER 39

Wellness Exams for Newborns, Infants, Children, and Adolescents

NEWBORNS AND INFANTS

What is a term infant?
A baby born between 37-weeks and 42-weeks gestation

Premature?
Less than 37 weeks

Postterm?
More than 42 weeks

When are Apgar scores measured?
At 1 and 5 minutes after birth

When should Apgar scores be repeated if the initial scores are less than 7?
At 10, 15, and 20 minutes after birth

What are the five Apgar categories?
1. Heart rate
2. Respiratory effort
3. Muscle tone
4. Reflex irritability
5. Color

What is the maximum number of points on the Apgar score?
There are up to 2 points in each category for a maximum of 10 points.

How many vessels does a normal umbilical cord have?
Three (two arteries and one vein)

How long does it typically take an umbilical cord stump to fall off?
1-3 weeks

How should the umbilical cord be maintained?	Air dry by keeping the diaper below the umbilicus; alcohol is not recommended; bathe the baby with a sponge bath but do not immerse the abdomen in water.
What is the typical weight of a healthy newborn?	2.5-4 kg
Length?	46-54 cm
Head circumference?	32-38 cm
What is the definition of low birth weight (LBW)?	Less than 2500 g at birth
What are the causes of LBW?	Intrauterine growth restriction (IUGR), prematurity, normal variant
What is the predominant cause of LBW in the United States?	Prematurity
What are the factors associated with IUGR (estimated fetal weight <10th percentile)?	Genetic abnormalities, multiple gestation, fetal insulin deficiency, placental insufficiency, maternal disease (eg, HTN, sickle cell disease), drug use
What is large for gestational age (LGA)?	Larger than 90th percentile for gestational age
What is the weight of a term LGA baby?	More than 4000 g
What is the most common cause of LGA babies?	Maternal diabetes
Normal newborns may lose up to what percentage of their weight in the first week of life?	Up to 10%
A healthy baby should regain this weight by how many weeks of life?	2 weeks
In the first couple of months, about how much weight should a baby gain per day?	1 oz (or 28 g)
A normal baby's respiratory rate and heart rate are slower than those of a normal adult. True or false?	False

A normal baby's blood pressure is lower than that of a normal adult. True or false?

True

Doing a good initial heart examination rules out heart abnormalities. True or false?

False

Why?

Some abnormalities may not be evident initially (eg, high pulmonary artery [PA] pressures on day one may diminish L → R shunting, so murmur of a ventral septal defect [VSD] is not appreciable)

When does the anterior fontanelle close?

During second year of life

Posterior fontanelle?

First few months of life

What is head "molding" in a newborn?

Irregularly shaped head with palpable ridges

What causes it?

Pressure in the birth canal during labor and delivery

How long does it normally last?

It should disappear within a week

What is caput succedaneum?

Diffuse soft tissue edema of the scalp

What causes it?

Pressure on presenting part of scalp during delivery

Does it require treatment?

No. It resolves on its own in a few days.

What is cephalohematoma?

Hemorrhage below the lining of the bones of the skull

What usually causes it?

Small tearing of vessels during delivery

What are worrisome causes?

Skull fracture, coagulopathy, intracerebral hemorrhage

What kind of treatment does an uncomplicated cephalohematoma require?

Usually none (resolves on its own), but the baby may need treatment for hyperbilirubinemia from blood resorption

Which crosses suture lines, cephalohematoma or caput succedaneum?

Caput succedaneum

What does an absent red reflex indicate?

Something is inhibiting light from getting to the retina (eg, cataract, tumor)

Intermittent strabismus is normal until what age?	3 months
What test on physical exam can assess ocular alignment?	The Hirschberg corneal light reflex test
How is the test performed?	The examiner notes the position of the corneal reflection from a light held 3 feet away from both eyes. Even with eye movement, the light should reflect in the same location of the cornea in each eye.
What will you see with left exotropia (left eye deviated laterally)?	The corneal reflection on the right will be over the pupil while the reflection on the left will be over the medial iris.
What is pseudostrabismus?	The perception of medial deviation (esotropia)
What contributes to pseudostrabismus?	Prominent medial canthal folds and a flat nasal bridge
What is the most common birth defect?	Hearing loss
What procedures are available to screen infants for hearing loss?	Measurement of otoacoustic emissions (OAEs) and/or auditory brain response (ABR)
All infants should be screened for hearing loss by what age?	1 month of age
Why is it so important to test for hearing loss?	Hearing loss can significantly delay a child's development, especially language acquisition.
Small, low-set, or floppy ears may be a sign of what other abnormalities?	Chromosomal abnormality, renal abnormality
A common benign newborn rash consisting of small white papules on a blotchy erythematous base is called what?	Erythema toxicum
What is the required treatment?	None (disappears on its own)
A female baby has swollen nipples and white vaginal discharge with a tinge of blood. Is this normal?	Yes
What is the cause?	Baby's exposure to maternal hormones

What is the American Academy of Pediatrics' stance on routine circumcision?	Not medically necessary
The Ortolani and Barlow maneuvers test for what abnormality?	Developmental hip dysplasia
What are some late diagnostic signs of developmental hip dysplasia?	Asymmetry of the following: thigh folds, hip abduction, and/or knee height
Lumbosacral dimples or hair tufts are concerning for what type of abnormality?	Underlying vertebral/spinal cord abnormality (eg, neural tube defect)
Does stroking the sole of the foot normally cause an infant's toes to go up or down?	Up
Stroking a newborn's cheek causes him to turn his head to the same side and make sucking motions with his mouth. What is this called?	Rooting reflex
When does the Moro reflex (startle reflex) normally disappear?	3-4 months
Every US state has a newborn screening program for metabolic and other inherited disorders. True or false?	True
Most state newborn screens include testing for what disorders?	Hypothyroidism, phenylketonuria, galactosemia, sickle cell disease
What is the most common chromosomal abnormality?	Down syndrome (Trisomy 21)
What are the most frequent causes of death in infants (<12 months old)?	Sudden infant death syndrome (SIDS), perinatal conditions (eg, complications of prematurity), congenital abnormalities, chromosomal abnormalities
About how many hours does a newborn sleep per 24 hours?	16-20 Tip: when you begin examining a newborn and s/he is not crying, take advantage of the opportunity to auscultate the heart and lungs and check for a red reflex.

INFANT FEEDING

When should breast-feeding begin?	Ideally, right after birth
What are the intrinsic benefits of breast milk compared to infant formula?	Composed of macro- and micronutrients specific and ideal for human babies, breast milk provides maternal antibodies (decreasing infections), is less expensive, and more environment friendly.
What additional benefits may be conferred to a breast-fed baby?	Decreased incidence of SIDS, lymphoma and other malignancies, obesity, diabetes, and allergies/eczema; increased IQ scores
What additional benefits of breast-feeding may be conferred to mothers?	Contracts uterus; helps in returning to prepregnancy weight; delay of menses; "Feel-good" hormone release (oxytocin); decreased incidence of breast cancer, ovarian cancer, and osteoporosis later in life
How often should a breast-fed infant feed?	8-12 times every 24 hours until 4 months of age
How long should each feeding last?	10-15 minutes on each breast
What is the current recommendation regarding breast-feeding in the developed world if the mother is HIV+?	Baby should be formula-fed because of risk for infection via breast milk.
How can we promote breast-feeding?	Education pre- and postdelivery about the benefits of breast-feeding, reinforcement, and early lactation training (proper latch-on techniques)
The American Academy of Pediatrics recommends breast-feeding for how long?	Exclusive breastfeeding for 6 months; then breastfeeding with appropriate complementary foods from 6 months to at least 12 months
What can be used as a supplement or alternative to breast milk?	Formula (cow-milk or soy-milk based)
The standard formula for a term infant has how many kilocalories per ounce?	20 kcal/oz

How many ounces should a formula-fed baby feed in the first few months of life?

On *average*, 2-3 oz every 3-4 hours by 2 weeks of age, progressively increasing to 5-6 oz every 3-4 hours at 6 months of age

How do you know if a baby is eating enough?

Plotting weight, length, and head circumference on a development curve

According to the American Academy of Pediatrics (AAP), what is the recommended daily intake of vitamin D for all infants, children, and adolescents?

400 International Units (IU) per day

What is the AAP's recommendation regarding vitamin D supplementation for breastfed and partially breastfed term infants?

The AAP recommends supplementing with 400 IU of vitamin D beginning in the first few days of life and continuing until the infant consumes at least 1 L per day (or 1 quart per day) of vitamin D-fortified formula or whole milk (though whole milk should not be used until after 12 months of age).

According to the AAP, what is the lower limit of normal for 25-hydroxyvitamin D concentrations in infants and children?

20 ng/mL

What is the USPSTF recommendation regarding screening for iron deficiency anemia?

There is insufficient evidence to recommend for/against routine screening for iron deficiency anemia in asymptomatic children aged 6-12 months (I recommendation). However, the USPSTF recommends routine iron supplementation (iron-fortified formula or iron supplements) for asymptomatic children aged 6-12 months who are at increased risk for iron deficiency anemia (B recommendation).

What are the sequelae of iron deficiency anemia in children?

Psychomotor and cognitive abnormalities, poor school performance

What are risk factors for iron deficiency anemia?

Prematurity, low birth weight infants

How early can you introduce solid foods to babies?

4 months

For how long may a baby's nutritional needs be met by formula or breast milk alone?	6 months
What are the signs that a baby is ready to eat solid foods?	Head control, loss of extrusion reflex, hunger that continues after consuming 32 oz of formula or nursing ten times per day
What types of food are appropriate for an infant beginning to eat solids?	Food that is soft and easy to digest (rice cereal with iron)
How should these foods be introduced?	Slowly and no more than one new food every 3 days (helps monitor for allergic reactions)
Do all babies spit up?	Generally, all babies will spit up at some time during feeds.
Why?	Babies have low esophageal sphincter tone, and caretakers frequently overfeed or inadequately burp them.
When is reflux worrisome?	Spitting up happens all of the time; weight gain is inadequate; reflux causes the baby to cry incessantly, cough, or wheeze
What should be the primary source of nutrition for a baby up to 1 year of age?	Breast milk or formula (solids are only a supplement)
What foods should be avoided in babies less than 12 months old?	Potent allergens such as egg whites, cow milk, honey, nut butters, citrus fruit, and seafood (especially shellfish)
Which of these can cause infant botulism poisoning?	Honey
What types of food should be avoided in children less than 3 years old?	Anything that may cause the toddler to choke (peanuts, whole grapes, raw vegetables that snap into hard chunks, etc)
What teeth are usually the first to erupt?	Mandibular central incisors
When (on average)?	6-8 months
What is the most common chronic childhood disease?	Dental caries
At what age should caregivers begin to clean a child's teeth?	As soon as the first teeth appear, a child's teeth can be cleansed with a cloth (later advancing to a soft toothbrush)

What is the USPSTF recommendation for fluoride supplementation?	The USPSTF recommends oral fluoride supplementation at recommended doses to preschool children older than 6 months of age whose primary water source is deficient in fluoride (B recommendation).
Which water sources have inconsistent levels of fluoride?	Well water and bottled water
Beginning at what age should a child's toothpaste contain fluoride?	2 years
Why is it important for young children to only use a small amount of fluorinated toothpaste and learn to rinse well and spit out as much toothpaste as possible when they are done brushing?	Swallowing large amounts of fluoride can cause a child's permanent teeth to have white spots.

JAUNDICE AND HYPERBILIRUBINEMIA

What is jaundice?	Yellowed skin and sclera secondary to increased levels of bilirubin
Where on the body can you first note jaundice and how does it then progress?	It starts in the gums and sclera, then progresses cephalocaudally. As bilirubin decreases, the jaundice recedes in the opposite direction.
Jaundice appears as a physical sign when bilirubin levels reach what approximate concentration?	5 mg/dL
What percent of term newborn infants have jaundice sometime during the first *week* of life?	60%
Premature newborns?	80%
Why is jaundice appearing within the first *day* of life so worrisome?	It is *always* pathologic
What is the differential diagnosis of jaundice on the first day of life?	Erythroblastosis fetalis, concealed hemorrhage, sepsis, intrauterine infection (eg, toxoplasmosis, rubella, cytomegalovirus [CMV], syphilis)

Describe physiologic jaundice of the newborn.

Breakdown of fetal RBCs + immature liver's inability to conjugate hemoglobin efficiently = jaundice secondary to rise in bilirubin

When does it peak?

Second to fourth day of life

When does it resolve?

Between fifth and seventh day

What clues might suggest that a newborn's jaundice is *not* physiologic?

Appears in the first 24-36 hours of life; bilirubin rises at >5 mg/dL per day, total is >12 mg/dL; jaundice lasts more than 10-14 days; conjugated bilirubin level is >1 mg/dL at any time (for some labs, it must also be >20% of the total bilirubin)

What is the fatal complication of hyperbilirubinemia?

Kernicterus

What is kernicterus?

Brain damage from unbound, unconjugated bilirubin crossing the blood brain barrier. It results in apoptosis and necrosis.

Which is neurotoxic, conjugated, or unconjugated bilirubin?

Unconjugated

At what level of total unconjugated bilirubin do you initiate treatment?

Depends on the newborn's age and risk factors, though generally between 11 mg/dL and 20 mg/dL

How is it most commonly treated?

Phototherapy

How does phototherapy work?

"Bili lights" are at a wavelength that converts bilirubin into a photoisomer that the body has an easier time excreting.

Describe breast-feeding failure jaundice versus breast milk jaundice.

Breast-feeding failure jaundice

This is an exaggeration of physiologic jaundice. It peaks within the first few days of life, is due to poor initial milk production and increased enterohepatic circulation, and is treated by increasing breast milk feedings.

Breast milk jaundice

It starts at 3-5 days, peaks at 2 weeks, and may be due to intrinsic factors in breast milk which increase the enterohepatic circulation.

GROWTH AND DEVELOPMENT

What three parameters should you plot on a growth chart at each well-child visit?	1. Weight and length 2. Height until adulthood 3. Head circumference the first 2 years
Why is it important to plot these values over time?	The overall pattern of growth (ie, *trajectory* of the curve) is more important than the raw values.
What are the most common causes of obesity in children?	Overeating and inactivity
Increased incidence of obesity has led to an increased incidence of what other diseases among children?	Type 2 diabetes mellitus, hypertension, hyperlipidemia
A BMI at what percentile defines a child as being overweight?	85th-95th (age-specific)
Obese?	Greater than 95th (age-specific)
What is failure to thrive (FTT)?	Inappropriately low weight (<3rd-5th percentile for the patient's age), growth curve that crosses two major percentiles, loss of weight
What accounts for 60%-80% of FTT?	Nonorganic and psychosocial causes (eg, poverty, neglect, mother with postpartum depression)
What are the organic causes of FTT?	Any medical condition that can cause inadequate caloric intake, absorption, or utilization (eg, gastroesophageal reflux disease [GERD], cystic fibrosis, food allergies, metabolic storage diseases); increased metabolic need (eg, congenital heart disease, chronic infection)
What is the treatment of FTT?	Frequent meals, increasing high-calorie solid food intake with additional supplementation if necessary, treatment of underlying medical condition

What are the benefits of assessing a child's physical, social, and cognitive development?	Delays are relatively easy to detect and give important information about a child's health
What is the Denver Developmental Screening Test?	A brief developmental assessment tool to screen 0-6 year olds
When assessing the development of a baby born prematurely, up until what age do you adjust his/her chronological age?	2 years
A nine-month-old baby who was born 3 months prematurely should be able to perform at what developmental level?	A 6-month-old

Approximately, at what age should a/n infant/child have the following gross motor skills?

While prone, lifts the head to 90°	3-4 months
Rolls front to back	4 months
Sits up with back unsupported	6 months
Crawls, cruises, and pulls to a stand	9 months
Takes first steps	12 months
Walks up the stairs supported by a wall or railing?	18 months
Runs well	2 years
Rides a tricycle	3 years

Approximately, at what age should a/n infant/child have the following fine motor skills?

Purposefully grasps an object	4-5 months
Pincer grasp	9 months
Copies a line	2 years
Copies a circle	3 years
Copies a square	4 years

Approximately, at what age should a/n
infant/child have the following
language skills?

Coos	2-3 months
Babbles	6 months
Says one or two distinct words	9-12 months
Follows one-step commands	12-15 months
Uses 2-3-word phrases	2 years
Speaks half intelligibly to a stranger	2 years
Speaks three-fourths intelligibly to a stranger	3 years
Speaks 100% intelligibly	4 years
Names four colors and four body parts	4 years

Approximately, at what age should a/n
infant/child have the following social
cognition skills?

Social smile	2 months
Laughs and squeals	4 months
Waves "bye-bye"	10 months
Plays alongside—but not with—other children (parallel play)	2 years
Plays with a group of other children	3 years

Approximately, over what ages do
Piaget stages of cognitive development
take place?

Sensorimotor (learns about the world through sensory perceptions and motor activities)	Birth-2 years
Preoperational (learns to use language, represent objects by symbols, but has difficulty taking the viewpoint of others)	2-7 years
Concrete operational (begins thinking logically about concrete events)	7-11 years
Formal operational (develops deductive reasoning, abstract thought, and systematic planning to solve problems)	11 years and older

On *average*, at what age do most babies begin to sleep 5-6 hours at a time?	6 months
When do stranger and separation anxiety usually begin?	7-9 months
When should toilet training begin in a child?	Every child is different, but usually between 18-30 months
Bed-wetting is normal up to what age?	4 years in girls and 5 years in boys

SAFETY AND PREVENTION

What general signs and symptoms of illness in a baby should parents learn to recognize?	Fever, poor feeding, decreased urine output, diarrhea, vomiting, inconsolable crying
What is the most common cause of death in children?	Unintentional injury
What bath safety tips should be given to all caregivers?	Set water heaters at lower than 120°F to prevent scalding burns and *never* leave children unattended
Why should infants be placed to sleep on their backs?	To help reduce the risk of sudden infant death syndrome (SIDS)
Infants/toddlers should ride in a rear facing infant or convertible car seat until what criteria are met?	At MINIMUM, until the child is 1 year old and weighs at least 20 pounds. Some manufacturers make seats that can safely remain rear facing beyond these criteria.
It is OK if caregivers smoke as long as it is only outdoors. True or false?	False. Smoking outdoors does not adequately eliminate second-hand smoking exposure.
Exposure to passive smoking has been linked to an increased incidence of what problems in infants and children?	Growth retardation, respiratory and ear infections, asthma, SIDS
You should not report child abuse unless you have a proof. True or false?	False. It is *mandatory* to report abuse, even if it is only a suspicion of abuse.

Overexposure to lead can have what significant health effects on children?	Low levels: behavior and cognitive problems (eg, learning disabilities) High levels: anemia, colic, nephropathy, encephalopathy, and even death
What is the USPSTF recommendation for lead screening?	There is insufficient evidence to recommend for/against screening in asymptomatic children aged 1-5 years who are at increased risk (I recommendation). The USPSTF recommends against screening asymptomatic children aged 1-5 years at average risk (D recommendation).
What factors can place a child at high-risk for lead exposure?	Living in or regularly visiting a house built before 1950, living in or regularly visiting a house built before 1978 that has had recent renovation (last 6 months), living near an industry that releases lead (such as a battery plant), exposure to lead glazed pottery, urban residence
What is a normal lead level (in µg/dL)?	No measurable level of lead is normal.

ADOLESCENTS

What do the Tanner Stages measure?	Sexual maturity
How many Tanner Stages are there?	Five
What is Tanner Stage 1?	Preadolescent
What is Tanner Stage 5?	Adult
What is the first visible sign of puberty in girls?	Appearance of breast buds, usually between 8-13 years
What physical changes follow?	Skeletal growth, pubic and axillary hair, menarche
When is menarche in relation to breast bud appearance?	About 2-2½ years later
What is the classic triad of McCune-Albright syndrome?	1. Polyostotic fibrous dysplasia 2. Café-au-lait spots 3. Precocious puberty

What is delayed sexual development in girls?

No breast development by the age of 14

What is primary amenorrhea?

No menarche by 16 years

What is the first visible sign of puberty in boys?

Testicular enlargement

What physical changes follow?

Pubic hair, enlargement of penis, spermarche, skeletal and muscle growth

What is delayed sexual development in boys?

No testicular enlargement by 16 years

What is the most common cause of delayed puberty?

Constitutional delay (a normal variant)

What labs do you use to evaluate delayed puberty if you suspect it is due to a disorder of the hypothalamic-pituitary-gonadal axis?

Follicle-stimulating hormone (FSH), luteinizing hormone (LH), estradiol (in girls) or testosterone (in boys)

What tests do you order if these are abnormal?

GnRH stimulation test and consider MRI to rule out cranial lesions

What is the most common chromosomal cause of delayed puberty in girls?

Turner syndrome (XO)—patients have gonadal dysgenesis

What physical examination findings may be seen in Turner syndrome?

Short stature, inner canthal folds with ptosis, short-webbed neck, widely spaced nipples, shield-like chest, lymphedema of the hands and feet

What are the three common cardiac defects associated with Turner syndrome?

1. Coarctation of the aorta
2. Bicuspid aortic valve
3. Aortic stenosis

What is the most common chromosomal cause of delayed puberty in boys?

Klinefelter syndrome (XXY)

What physical examination findings are seen in Klinefelter syndrome?

Tall stature with a height : arm span ratio of >1, small testes/penis, gynecomastia

What are the characteristics of Kallmann syndrome?

Hypogonadotropic hypogonadism, anosmia or hyposmia, delayed puberty, small penis in boys, lack of breast development in girls

When evaluating an adolescent, what does the acronym "HEADSS" stand for?

Home, education and employment, activity, drugs, sexuality, and suicide and depression

What is the significance of the "HEADSS" mnemonic?

Builds a rapport; obtains information about risk exposure; guides preventive measures, including education on sensitive topics

What are the top three causes of death among adolescents?

1. Unintentional injury/trauma
2. Homicide
3. Suicide

CHAPTER 40

Geriatric Wellness

A person's ability or inability to perform ADLs (activities of daily living) and IADLs (instrumental activities of daily living) determines functional status. What are some examples of ADLs?

Eating, grooming, dressing, toileting, control of bowel and bladder function, transferring from bed to chair

Examples of IADLs?

Transportation, shopping, managing finances, cooking, cleaning/laundry, using the telephone, taking medications accurately

Why is it important to assess an elderly patient's functional status?

Understanding a patient's functional status helps determine what kind of support s/he needs in order to remain as safe, satisfied, and as independent as possible.

What problems lead to decrease in functional status?

Hearing/vision loss, dementia, depression, malnutrition, age-related physical changes as well as medical and dental disease-related changes, medications

What is presbycusis?

Hearing loss associated with aging (usually sensorineural)

What are the symptoms of presbycusis?

Difficulty understanding speech, sounds seem less clear and lower in volume (high-pitched sounds are particularly difficult to discern), some sounds seem overly loud and annoying (hyperacusis), tinnitus

What is the most common cause of presbycusis?

Repeated exposure to loud noises over time

How is presbycusis treated?

There is no cure for presbycusis; however, hearing aids prove to be beneficial for many patients.

What are the causes of ear canal obstruction and subsequent *conductive* hearing loss?

Cerumen impaction (most common), foreign bodies (cotton swab tip, insect), tumors

What is presbyopia?

Vision loss associated with aging

What are some other conditions that lead to vision loss in the elderly?

Diabetic retinopathy, macular degeneration, glaucoma, cataracts

For what reasons does dental disease pose a threat to an elderly person's functional status?

Dental problems (missing teeth, loose dentures, gum/tooth pain, etc) can lead to problems with eating (which can then contribute to malnutrition) and problems with speaking (which can contribute to social isolation).

Memory loss is a normal part of aging. True or false?

False

What is dementia?

It is impaired memory and cognitive function without an alteration in consciousness. It interferes with normal daily functioning and may cause changes in mood, behavior, and personality.

Name some easy and inexpensive tests that can be used to help diagnose dementia.

Folstein mini-mental status exam, clock test

What is the most common cause of dementia?

Alzheimer dementia

What classes of medications are used to treat Alzheimer dementia?

Cholinesterase inhibitors (donepezil, rivastigmine, galantamine) and NMDA receptor antagonist (Memantine)

What is the second most common cause of dementia?

Vascular (multiinfarct) dementia

What is pseudodementia?

Depression that causes memory and cognitive disturbance

What is the geriatric depression scale?

A 30-item "yes or no" questionnaire used to help diagnose depression in the elderly

What treatable vitamin deficiency may cause a cognitive disturbance as well as macrocytic anemia?

Vitamin B_{12} deficiency

What treatable endocrine abnormality may cause cognitive disturbance as well as fatigue, bradycardia, constipation, and cold intolerance?

Hypothyroidism

What sexually transmitted illnesses can lead to cognitive disturbances?

AIDS and syphilis (neurosyphilis)

What disease causes a triad of dementia, gait disturbance, and urinary incontinence? (Hint: a CT scan is helpful in the diagnosis.)

Normal pressure hydrocephalus

Name some other chronic conditions (not mentioned so far) that may cause dementia symptoms.

Parkinson disease, Lewy body dementia, chronic alcohol abuse, medication misuse or medication side effects, metabolic disturbances (eg, hyponatremia—usually acute, but can also develop over time)

Acute altered mental status (AMS) can present in patients of all age groups, but can present an especially confusing clinical picture in patients who have baseline dementia. What are the causes of AMS?

(Here is one version of the mnemonic AEIOU TIP…)

A = Alcohol, Arterial occlusion or rupture, Adrenal insufficiency

E = Electrolyte disturbances, Endocrinopathies, Encephalopathy, Embolus

I = Insulin (hypoglycemia), Inflammation (vasculitis)

O = drug Overdose, Oxygen (hypoxia)

U = Uremia

T = Trauma (especially to the head), Toxins, Temperature (fever or hypothermia), Thyroid disease

I = severe Infections (meningitis, sepsis), renal Insufficiency

P = Psychiatric problems, Pulmonary problems (embolus, hypercarbia, hypoxia), poor Pump (heart failure)

S = Seizures, Stroke, Shock, Space occupier (tumor, hemorrhaged blood)

If incontinence is affecting a patient, s/he is likely to bring it up during a routine physical exam; therefore, it is not necessary for a health care provider to ask about incontinence since questioning the patient may embarrass her/him. True or false?

False! Screening for incontinence should be a part of a routine physical.

What is the recommended geriatric vaccination schedule for the following?

Td	Td booster every 10 years
Varicella	Two doses for patients without evidence of immunity
Shingles	A single dose for patients 60 years and older regardless of whether they report a history of shingles
Influenza	One dose annually after age 50
Pneumococcal	One dose for patients 65 years and older, with a repeat dose 5 years later

Why is it so important to assess geriatric patients' risk for falling? — The complications arising from fall injuries are a leading cause of preventable morbidity and mortality amongst the elderly

What factors increase a patient's likelihood to fall? — Decreased vision, orthostatic hypotension, decreased muscle strength and coordination, dizziness, and other medication side effects

What are some simple screening methods for malnutrition? — Charting a patient's weight over several visits, asking caregivers about changes in appetite

What is the recommended daily dose of vitamin D for people over the age of 50 years? — 800-1000 IU per day (but up to 2000 IU is ok)

What is the recommended daily dose of calcium for the following groups?

Men aged 50-65 years	1000 mg
Women aged 50-65 years who are on estrogen replacement therapy	1000 mg
Men and women over 65 years old	1200-1500 mg

What is the most common gastrointestinal side effect of calcium carbonate? — Constipation

What preparations of calcium do not tend to cause constipation? — Calcium citrate and calcium phosphate

What is the Beers criteria? — It is an expert-compiled list of potentially inappropriate medications for the elderly because of the adverse side effects they could cause.

Most people over what age are eligible for Medicare?

65

What does Medicare Part A cover?

Hospital stays as well as posthospital nursing and home health

What does Medicare Part B cover?

Most basic outpatient services (doctor visits, labs, supplies and equipment, home health care, physical therapy)

What does Medicare Part D cover?

Some prescription medications

What is durable power of attorney?

A person that has been designated by a patient as his/her surrogate decision maker in the event that s/he can no longer make decisions

What are advance directives?

Written or oral statements that a *competent* patient makes in order that their family and health care providers may provide care according to his/her wishes should the patient become incompetent

What does DNR stand for?

Do not resuscitate

CHAPTER 41

Preparticipation Sports Physical

85% of deaths in young athletes are due to underlying abnormalities of what organ system?

Cardiovascular system

What eight history questions are key to evaluating the young athlete's cardiovascular history?

Has the patient had the following:

1. Exertional chest pain?
2. Unexplained syncope or presyncope?
3. Excessive dyspnea or fatigue?
4. A heart murmur?
5. Elevated blood pressure (BP)?
6. A 1st or 2nd degree family member that died before age 50 due to heart disease?
7. A 1st or 2nd degree family member who had disability from heart disease before age 50?
8. A family member with hypertrophic cardiomyopathy, long QT syndrome, Marfan syndrome, or other cardiomyopathy or rhythm abnormality?

What four physical exam findings are key to screening for heart disease in an athlete?

Does the patient have the following:

1. Heart murmur?
2. Equal femoral pulses?
3. Physical stigmata of Marfan syndrome?
4. Brachial artery high BP?

A patient with highly arched palate, scoliosis, pes planus, arachnodactyly, mitral valve prolapse, arm span-to-height ratio >1.05, and pectus excavatum would make you concerned for what disorder?

Marfan syndrome

Patients with Marfan syndrome are at risk for what cardiovascular problems?

Valvular disorders and aortic dilation leading to dissection or rupture

What skin conditions should be treated prior to clearance for participation in close contact sports?

Molluscum contagiosum, tinea corporis, and herpes gladiatorum

The physical exam consists of what steps?

HEENT—check vision, examine pupil size, examine nares and ears (for water sports)

CV—auscultate the heart supine and standing, as well as with a dynamic maneuver or Valsalva; palpate femoral pulses

RESP—auscultate lungs

ABD—examine abdomen for organomegaly

GU (males)—check for two testicles and presence of masses or hernias

SKIN—assess skin condition

MUSC—assess strength and mobility of joints

NEURO—brief neurologic exam

What is the range for a healthy body mass index (BMI)?

BMI >19 kg/m^2 and <25 kg/m^2

An enhanced preseason conditioning program should be considered for what patients?

BMI >25 kg/m^2

A patient with one testicle should be told the following in regards to sports participation.

Needs to wear protection over scrotum during sporting events

A murmur that is systolic, increases with standing and Valsalva, and decreases with squatting and a supine position is indicative of what underlying disorder?

Hypertrophic cardiomyopathy (HCM)

What cardiac murmurs require further evaluation prior to clearance for sports?

Diastolic murmur, systolic murmur 3/6 or greater, or murmur with characteristics of HCM

In addition to murmurs, what other cardiac findings require further evaluation prior to clearance?

Tachycardia, severe hypertension in a child, or stage II hypertension in an adult

What should you do with an athlete with corrected vision 20/50 or worse in one eye?

Send for further evaluation and clear only if wearing full eye protection during athletic activities

The female athlete triad consists of what findings?

Disordered eating, amenorrhea, and osteopenia or osteoporosis

Contact sports are contraindicated for patients with what chronic conditions?

Solitary functional kidney, atlantoaxial instability, hepatomegaly, splenomegaly, poorly controlled seizure disorder

An enlarged spleen is a contraindication for clearance and suggestive of what underlying disease process?

Infectious mononucleosis

A history of numbness or weakness that occurs simultaneously in more than one extremity is suggestive of what underlying condition and should be evaluated prior to clearance?

Cervical cord neuropraxia

A traction or compression injury to the nerves of the brachial plexus or cervical roots is commonly called by what name?

A "stinger" or "burner," also known as transient neuropraxia

A patient who is asymptomatic at rest but complains of symptoms of cough, chest tightness, or loss of endurance with exercise suggests what diagnosis?

Exercise-induced asthma (EIA)

CHAPTER 42

Domestic Violence

When is reporting of domestic violence mandatory?	Specific reporting laws vary by state, but in all states, reporting is mandatory if the victim is under the age of 18 or over the age of 60. Some states mandate reporting for all victims.
How is domestic violence reported?	Each state has a direct phone line and/or Internet link to report abuse to that state's appropriate government department (eg, Department of Homeland Security, Department of Health, Department of Family and Protective Services).
How does abuse affect the health of the victim?	Complications from physical injuries (including death), disruption of normal immune function, disruption of normal sleep, increased risk of certain psychosocial and medical conditions (eg, depression, developmental delays, heart disease, cancer)
What psychiatric disorders are more common in a patient who is a victim of violence?	Substance abuse, anxiety, depression, eating disorders
Victims of abuse often report what somatic complaints?	Chronic pain (abdominal, pelvic), headaches, fatigue

What conditions place a person at a higher risk for violence victimization?

- High-need situations: young or old age, pregnancy, disease, or disabilities
- Caregivers are uneducated and/or have little understanding of the victim's needs
- Caregivers are under increased significant stress: single parenthood, unemployment
- Residence in a violent and/or low-income community
- For children, having nonbiological caregivers in the home

What are the four types of child maltreatment?

1. Physical abuse: causing intentional injury to victim's body (eg, hitting, biting, pushing, drugging, inappropriate restraint)
2. Sexual abuse: using any body part to touch (directly or through clothing) a child's breasts, buttocks, and/or genitalia for sexual pleasure (or coercing the child to touch perpetrator in this manner). Any kind of sexual exploitation (eg, exhibitionism, pornography). Intentionally exposing child to sexual acts.
3. Emotional abuse: speaking or acting (or withholding speech or acts) in such a way that demoralizes, demeans, threatens, intimidates, or unfairly blames or criticizes the victim
4. Neglect: failure to provide adequate supervision, intentional exposure to unsafe environment, failure to provide basic needs (food and shelter, emotional support and affection, safety, medical and dental care, education)

What are the six types of elder maltreatment?

1. Physical abuse
2. Sexual abuse: any sexual act done without competent consent
3. Emotional abuse
4. Neglect
5. Abandonment: intentionally deserting and leaving elder without a responsible caregiver
6. Financial abuse: illegal and/or unethical use of elder's assets

What are the four main types of intimate partner violence?

1. Physical abuse
2. Sexual abuse
3. Threats of physical or sexual violence
4. Psychological/emotional violence

Why are physical signs from abuse not always evident when a health care provider examines the victim?

The abusive acts may have not caused physically visible harm (emotional abuse, sexual acts done through touching) or time elapses and physically visible injuries heal between the time of perpetration and reporting of abuse.

What are some questions you can ask to screen for domestic violence?

- Do you feel safe in your relationship?
- Have you ever been in a relationship where you were threatened, hurt, or afraid?
- Are your friends or family aware that you have been hurt?
- Could you tell them and would they be able to give you support?
- Do you have a safe place to go and the resources you need in an emergency?

CHAPTER 43

Travel Medicine

What is the leading cause of death among older persons traveling abroad?	Coronary artery disease
What is the leading cause of death among younger persons traveling abroad?	Trauma. Accidents (especially motor vehicle accidents) account for one-fourth of deaths among Americans abroad.
What is the definition of classic traveler's diarrhea?	Passage of three or more unformed stools (occasionally explosive) in a 24-hour period plus at least one of these symptoms: nausea, vomiting, abdominal pain, fever, tenesmus, or blood in stool
What percentage of those traveling to developing countries will get traveler's diarrhea?	40%-60%
What is the most common pathogen implicated in traveler's diarrhea?	Enterotoxigenic *Escherichia coli* (ETEC)
Which food and water precautions can decrease the likelihood of developing traveler's diarrhea?	Peel fruit with clean utensils. Avoid raw vegetables (eg, lettuce), ice from unclean water, unpasteurized dairy products, and inadequately cooked meat or fish. Purify water (with boiling, chlorine, iodine, or filtration systems) that may be contaminated.
The majority of traveler's diarrhea is self-limited. True or false?	True, though dehydration can complicate an episode and antibiotics can decrease the duration of symptoms by one day
What is the typical time course for traveler's diarrhea?	Symptoms last 1-5 days, start between 4 and 14 days after arrival, can appear within 10 days after the patient returns home

Which antibiotics can be used to treat moderate to severe traveler's diarrhea (characterized by fever; four or more unformed stools daily; blood, pus, or mucus in the stool)?	Ciprofloxacin 500 mg PO twice daily for 1-2 days (though other quinolones can also be used), azithromycin 1 g PO × 1 (particularly given increasing resistance to quinolones), rifaximin 200 mg PO three times daily
Bismuth subsalicylate can be used for the treatment and prevention of traveler's diarrhea. True or false?	True
Which malaria prophylaxis medication is not well absorbed when administered concurrently with bismuth subsalicylate?	Doxycycline
Which activity increases the risk of acquiring schistosomiasis?	Swimming or walking in unchlorinated freshwater areas where schistosomiasis is prevalent
What are symptoms of high altitude illness?	Headache, fatigue, lightheadedness, anorexia, nausea/vomiting, disturbed sleep with frequent awakening, mild shortness of breath with exertion
What measures can treat high altitude illness?	Descent to a lower altitude, oxygen, dexamethasone
What measures can decrease the risk of developing high altitude illness?	Gradual ascent, preexposure to higher altitudes, alcohol and sedative avoidance, acetazolamide
Which vaccines are required for travel?	The live yellow fever vaccine is required for entry into certain countries. For travelers to Saudi Arabia during the Hajj, the tetravalent meningococcal vaccine (administered not more than 3 years and not less than 10 days before arrival) is required for all travelers, and infants and children up to 15 years of age need documentation of polio vaccination.
Which vaccines may be recommended depending on immunity status, geographic region, and season of travel?	Polio, tetanus, measles, typhoid, rabies, hepatitis A, hepatitis B, influenza, meningococcus, Japanese encephalitis, tick-borne encephalitis (vaccine not available in the United States)

Which insect repellant should be recommended to all travelers at risk for vector borne diseases?

DEET, 30%

What other measures can reduce exposure to vector borne diseases?

Clothing that reduces the amount of exposed skin, using permethrin-impregnated bed nets in high-risk areas, avoiding outdoor exposure between dusk and dawn when *Anopheles* mosquitoes feed, malaria chemoprophylaxis

Which medications are indicated for malaria chemoprophylaxis?

Atovaquone-proguanil, mefloquine, doxycycline, chloroquine, primaquine

Which medication(s) can prevent development of hepatic hypnozoite forms?

Primaquine

What percentage of travelers is not compliant with malaria prophylaxis?

50%-60%. Chemoprophylaxis is typically started prior to travel and continued regularly during exposure and for a period of time following departure.

For more specific information about required and recommended vaccinations and malaria risk and resistance, consult www.cdc.gov/travel or www.who.int/ith/en/

CHAPTER 44

Basic Obstetrical Care

How soon after conception can a urine pregnancy test be positive?

The test may be positive as soon as 1 week after conception

What hormone do pregnancy tests detect?

Beta-human chorionic gonadotrophin (beta-hCG)

Urine and pregnancy tests can detect pregnancy at what level of beta-hCG?

Urine: 20-50 mIU/mL

Serum: 5 mIU/mL

In the first weeks of a normal pregnancy, approximately how often does beta-hCG double?

Approximately every 2 days

What are the two most common causes of a faster than normal beta-hCG rise?

1. Multiple gestation
2. Molar pregnancy

What are the two most common causes of a slower than normal beta-hCG rise?

1. Impending miscarriage
2. Ectopic pregnancy

What are the most common symptoms of a spontaneous abortion?

Abdominal cramping and vaginal bleeding

What is the most common cause of spontaneous abortions?

Chromosomal abnormality (usually trisomy)

Perinatal infections account for about 3% of all congenital anomalies. The most common ones are known as the TORCH infections. Name these.

- Toxoplasmosis
- Other (syphilis, varicella, parvovirus B19)
- Rubella
- Cytomegalovirus
- Herpes

Why should pregnant women avoid changing cat litter?

Cat feces may contain the parasite *Toxoplasma gondii*, the etiologic agent of toxoplasmosis.

Why are the food-borne illnesses listeria, toxoplasmosis, campylobacter, and salmonella, particularly dangerous for pregnant women?

They can cause severe fetal disease, stillbirth, or miscarriage.

Can women be vaccinated for varicella and rubella during pregnancy?

No

What is the most common cause of preventable mental retardation?

Alcohol, which causes the spectrum of abnormalities called fetal alcohol syndrome disorders. Women should be advised that no amount of alcohol is safe during pregnancy.

What class of common over-the-counter pain medications is not advised in pregnancy due to potential premature closure of the ductus arteriosus?

Nonsteroidal anti-inflammatory drugs (NSAIDs)

What does it mean when the Food and Drug Administration (FDA) labels a prescription drug as "X"?

The drug is contraindicated in pregnancy because any potential benefit to the mother does not outweigh the potential harm to the fetus (eg, isotretinoin for acne).

What does the FDA's drug label "A" mean?

There are *human* studies demonstrating the drug's safety in pregnancy

For a routine pregnancy, what is the recommended dosage of folic acid during the early prenatal period and why is it an important supplement?

Taking 400 µg daily beginning 3 months before conception helps prevent neural tube defects

What is the recommended daily dose of calcium for pregnant and lactating women?

1200-1500 mg

What is the beta-hCG threshold at which transvaginal ultrasound should reveal an intrauterine pregnancy?

1500 mIU/mL

What is the most likely diagnosis when beta-hCG is above 1500 mIU/mL but there is no pregnancy seen on ultrasound?

Ectopic pregnancy

When can fetal heart tones be heard using transabdominal Doppler beginning at how many weeks gestation?

9-12 weeks

In general, for healthy women presenting for an initial prenatal care office visit, what labs and tests should be performed?

Blood type/Rh and antibody screen (ABO/Rh), hemoglobin and hematocrit, rubella titer, syphilis screen, hepatitis B surface antigen, HIV, chlamydia, gonorrhea, cystic fibrosis carrier screening, varicella immunity screening, Pap smear, urine analysis and culture

Why is a urinalysis routinely ordered in pregnant women?

Urinalysis helps detect asymptomatic urinary tract infections as well as screen for proteinuria (may indicate development of preeclampsia)

The lab test (done between 11 and 14 weeks gestation) which measures the blood levels of pregnancy-associated plasma protein-A (PAPP-A) and hCG along with ultrasound-guided nuchal translucency screening helps detect what genetic condition(s)?

Down syndrome and Trisomy 18

What is the significance of the following second and third trimester labs?

"Quad screen" (aka "multiple marker screening"): alpha fetoprotein (AFP), estriol, free beta-hCG, inhibin-A (15-20-weeks gestation)

Helps detect Down syndrome, Trisomy 18, and neural tube defects; a patient with an abnormal result may be referred for further testing (amniocentesis, ultrasound). See the table Quad Screen Interpretation

Quad Screen Interpretation

	Alpha Fetoprotein (AFP)	Estriol	Free Beta-hCG	Inhibin-A
Down syndrome	↓	↓	↑	↑
Trisomy 18	↓	↓	↓	
Neural tube defects	↑			

One-hour glucose challenge (24-28-weeks gestation)

Helps detect gestational diabetes. Test performed during the first trimester and repeated in the second trimester, if patient has risk factors for gestational diabetes. An abnormal result should be followed up by a 3-hour glucose challenge.

Group B *streptococcus* culture (35-37-weeks gestation)

If positive, the patient will require antibiotics during labor to avoid transmitting GBS to baby during vaginal delivery. GBS is the leading cause of life-threatening infection in newborns.

Why is it particularly important for women to receive dental care during pregnancy?	At least 50% of pregnant women have gum disease (due to hormonal changes and decreased ability to fight infection). Severe gum disease has been linked to intrauterine growth retardation and preterm labor.
What drug is used to prevent maternal sensitization to Rh D antigens?	RhoGAM
Is RhoGAM given to mothers who are Rh negative or positive?	Negative
When is RhoGAM given?	Once at 28-30-weeks gestation, then again soon after delivery, if the baby is Rh positive; also given with trauma, bleeding, and spontaneous abortion
What are the categories of hypertension (HTN) in pregnancy?	Chronic HTN, preeclampsia, chronic HTN with superimposed preeclampsia, gestational HTN
What is preeclampsia?	New onset of HTN (systolic BP >140 mm Hg or diastolic BP >90 mm Hg) and proteinuria (24-hour urine protein is $\geq$0.3 g) after 20-weeks gestation
What kind of pregnancy is suspected if preeclampsia symptoms present before 20 weeks of gestation?	Molar pregnancy
What are common risk factors for preeclampsia?	Nulliparity; multiple gestations; teenager or age >35 years; African American or Hispanic race; personal or family history of preeclampsia; chronic HTN; vascular, renal, or immune disease; obesity; diabetes
What is the most common neurologic symptom of preeclampsia?	Headache
What are the signs and symptoms of severe preeclampsia?	Headache, confusion, blurred or double vision, nausea and vomiting, right upper quadrant or epigastric pain, oliguria, hematuria, fetal distress, placental abruption
What is HELLP syndrome?	A severe form of preeclampsia in which a patient develops **H**emolysis, **E**levated **L**iver enzymes, and **L**ow **P**latelets

What is eclampsia?

The development of seizures in a preeclamptic patient, often preceded by a headache

What is the definitive treatment for preeclampsia/eclampsia?

Delivery of the fetus

What medication is used to prevent seizures in preeclampsia?

Magnesium sulfate

What is gestational HTN?

HTN that develops after 20-weeks gestation without any other features of preeclampsia; resolves within 12 weeks postpartum

What hypertensive medications are generally safe to use in pregnancy?

Labetalol, methyldopa, nifedipine, and hydralazine

What are Braxton-Hicks contractions?

Irregular, painless (or only mildly cramping) contractions that occur beginning about the 6th week of pregnancy, but are usually not noticed until the second and third trimester

If a laboring patient presents with vaginal bleeding, what should you do before doing a digital pelvic exam?

Ultrasound to rule out placenta previa

What are the absolute contraindications for vaginal delivery?

Placenta previa, active herpes simplex infection (or prodromal symptoms), history of uterine surgery involving the active portion of the uterus (eg, cesarean delivery with classic incision), untreated HIV infection

For routine labor management, what is the purpose of serial pelvic exams?

Assess cervical change (dilation, effacement, consistency, position), station, fetal presentation and fetal position; if relevant, verify rupture of membranes (with sterile speculum). Initial exam should assess adequacy of pelvis.

The presenting part is said to be at 0 station when it is at the level of what bony structure?

The mother's ischial spines

What is premature rupture of membranes (PROM)?

Rupture of membranes before the initiation of labor

What are the ways of confirming rupture of membranes?	Sterile speculum exam shows pooling and leakage of fluid with Valsalva; microscopic examination of fluid is nitrazine positive and reveals ferning under the microscope
What are the components of the Bishop scoring system used to predict the success of a labor induction?	Dilation, effacement, station, consistency, position of cervix
Cervical ripening should be considered at what Bishop score?	Less than 6
What is the definition of labor?	Cervical change (dilation, effacement), accompanied by regular uterine contractions
What is the definition of preterm labor?	Labor that occurs before 37-weeks gestation
What are the risk factors for preterm labor?	Multiple gestations, history of preterm labor, uterine and cervical abnormalities (eg, fibroids, cervical incompetence)
What are the stages of labor?	First stage: latent phase (up to 4 cm dilation) and active phase (from 4-10 cm dilation)
	Second stage: complete dilation of the cervix to delivery of infant
	Third stage: delivery of infant to delivery of placenta
What is the range of normal baseline fetal heart rate?	110-160 beats per minute
Fetal heart rate variability should be normal after how many weeks gestation?	After 32 weeks
What type of deceleration is associated with umbilical cord compression?	Variable deceleration
What type of deceleration is associated with uteroplacental insufficiency (leading to fetal hypoxia or acidemia in severe cases)?	Late decelerations

What type of deceleration is associated with fetal head compression during uterine contractions?

Early decelerations

What are the three "P's" that you should assess when a patient has a labor dystocia?

1. Passenger (fetus: size, presentation, position)
2. Power (contractions, maternal expulsive force)
3. Passage/pelvis (bony anatomy and soft tissues)

What are the seven cardinal movements that describe the changes in position of the fetal head as it passes through the birth canal?

1. Engagement
2. Descent
3. Flexion
4. Internal rotation
5. Extension
6. External rotation
7. Expulsion

What is puerperium?

The 6-8-week period postpartum when the body gradually returns to its nonpregnant state

What is lochia?

Vaginal discharge immediately after delivery from blood clots expelled from the uterus and decidua that gradually sloughs off

How long does it take for the uterus to return to its prepregnancy size?

6-8 weeks

When does ovulation resume in nonbreast-feeding women?

On average, 10 weeks after delivery

When does ovulation resume in breast-feeding women?

For some women, ovulation is unaffected by breastfeeding; in others, it resumes after weaning. On average, nursing mothers resume menses between 6 months and 2 years postpartum.

In the United States, what are the contraindications to breast-feeding?

Mother with HIV or HTLV-1 (human T-cell lymphotropic virus), history of drug abuse, or is taking antineoplastic or antimetabolic drugs; infant with galactosemia

What is breast engorgement?

Swelling of the breast from edema and/or accumulated milk

What are common infections during the postpartum period?

Endometritis, UTI, mastitis, wound infection, pelvic thrombophlebitis

Vaccination against what diseases should be given to all nonimmune postpartum patients, including breast-feeding mothers, if there are no contraindications?

Rubella (component of MMR), varicella, pertussis (component of Tdap), influenza (seasonal)

What are postpartum baby blues and how common are they?

Baby blues occur in about three-fourths of women and are characterized by feelings of sadness and anxiety, tearfulness, trouble sleeping, and eating.

How do baby blues differ from postpartum depression?

Baby blues are transitory and usually resolve within a week without treatment. Most importantly, they do not interfere with normal functioning. The mother is able to care for herself and her infant.

What percentage of mothers has postpartum depression?

About 10%

What is the first-line treatment for postpartum depression?

Cognitive behavioral therapy and antidepressants (usually selective serotonin reuptake inhibitor, such as sertraline)

SECTION V
Clinical Vignettes

CHAPTER 45

Clinical Vignettes

1. A 56-year-old White male comes to your clinic for a physical examination and you give him a clean bill of health. He is normotensive. A few years later the same patient comes back and is overweight with a blood pressure (BP) of 135/85 mm Hg (subsequently confirmed). The rest of the examination is normal.

   What is your diagnosis?

   Prehypertension

   What lifestyle modifications would you recommend?

   Weight reduction, dietary approaches to stop hypertension (HTN) (DASH) diet, physical activity, no more than 1 oz of alcohol per day

   If this patient later develops HTN, but has no other comorbidities, what would be your first line of drug therapy?

   Thiazide diuretic

2. A 65-year-old Hispanic male comes in for his yearly examination and appears healthy. Review of systems is negative. He is retired, eats well, and plays tennis three times a week. Body mass index (BMI) = 24 kg/m². When he was 60 years old he had a colonoscopy showing no abnormalities.

   Assuming he remains asymptomatic, when should he repeat colon cancer screening?

   Age 70

   For what other diseases would you screen this patient?

   Hyperlipidemia, HTN, alcohol misuse, depression

   If the patient has HTN, for what other disease would you screen this patient?

   Diabetes mellitus

   If the patient tells you he smoked one pack of cigarettes a week for one year when he was in his forties, what other screening(s) would you do?

   Screen for abdominal aortic aneurysm with abdominal ultrasonography

3. **A 48-year-old obese female comes into the office stating that her right hip has been hurting for a couple of weeks and she cannot sleep on her right side. The rest of her review of systems is noncontributory. Upon examination, the patient has point tenderness over the greater trochanter, but otherwise has a normal exam.**

What is the most likely initial diagnosis?

Nonseptic trochanteric bursitis

What physical examination findings could be indicative of a more serious condition?

Signs of infection, such as fever or overlying skin changes

Is this patient truly experiencing pain in her *hip* joint?

The hip joints (which are affected in diseases like osteoarthritis [OA]) attach to the pelvis in the *groin*. Her pain is over the greater trochanteric bursa along the lateral thigh. Patients often mistakenly complain of "hip pain" with bursitis and "groin pain" with OA.

Assuming that you decide to treat the patient with a corticosteroid shot, is aspiration prior to the shot indicated, and if so, why?

No. While it is a good idea to aspirate superficial bursa with obvious swelling and/or infection, aspiration at deep bursae yield little to no fluid and only causes patient discomfort.

4. **A 65-year-old female complains of a 7-month history of knee pain and stiffness, worse at the end of the day. She has also been noticing pain in her hips, back, and hands, particularly at the base of the thumbs.**

What is the most likely diagnosis?

OA

You notice a square appearance of the radial aspect of her hands. What is this finding called?

Shelf sign

What is the most *specific* radiographic marker for OA?

Osteophytes

Why is exercise important for this patient?

Exercise prevents muscle spasm and atrophy; promotes weight loss; and ideally, postpones the need for surgery

What kind of exercise would you recommend?

Minimize weight-bearing exercises. Swimming is ideal.

5. **A 40-year-old male with HTN presents with complaint of colicky abdominal pain, nausea, and hematuria for the last day. He had been working outside in his yard all weekend and had not been drinking a lot of water.**

What are two possible basic imaging tests used to detect the suspected diagnosis?

1. Abdominal plain film (KUB)
2. Intravenous pyelography (IVP)

What imaging test has become the gold standard, and can be considered, if stones are not detected on the above imaging tests?

Noncontrast helical CT scan

What is the imaging test of choice in a patient who cannot be exposed to radiation?

Ultrasonography

What is the initial management of a patient with renal colic?

Pain control with NSAIDs and/or opioids, hydration, and straining urine

A stone less than what diameter is likely to pass spontaneously?

Less than 4 mm

80% of patients with urolithiasis form stones composed of what mineral?

Calcium (calcium oxalate or calcium phosphate)

A history of obesity, chronic diarrhea, or gout makes you concerned for what type of stone?

Uric acid stone

What elements in the presentation would necessitate metabolic workup for causes of stones?

Multiple stones on initial presentation, family history of stones, recurrent stone formation

6. A young adult male complains of fever for 1 week, sore throat, and fatigue. He had unprotected sex 3 weeks ago, and later admits that he has had unprotected sex "several times" in the last year. Examination: T 38°C, cervical lymphadenopathy, supple neck, faint macular rash, pharyngitis with exudates, splenomegaly.

What tests would you order to aid in your initial diagnosis?

Complete blood count (CBC)

Monospot test

Throat culture (include testing for gonorrhea and chlamydia)

HIV viral load test

In the setting of acute HIV infection, why can you not rely on an ELISA or a Western blot test alone to make the diagnosis?

These tests can be negative in the acute phase.

7. A 65-year-old male complains of squeezing chest pain that radiates to his jaw. Episodes last two minutes, are brought on by exercise, and relieved with rest. The pain is not associated with food intake and not relieved by antacids. He denies fever, diaphoresis, dyspnea, and nausea.

What is the *most likely* diagnosis?

Stable angina resulting from ischemic heart disease

What tests help you rule out a myocardial infarction (MI)?

Cardiac enzymes, electrocardiogram

Assuming that the MI workup is negative, what noninvasive test would you use to assess the degree of ischemic heart disease?

Exercise stress test

What medications are available to treat anginal pain?

Nitrates, beta-blockers, calcium-channel blockers

8. **A 50-year-old male presents for his annual well exam. After taking a thorough history, examining the patient, and obtaining the appropriate labs, you diagnose the patient with type II diabetes mellitus and HTN. His kidney function is normal.**

What is the BP goal for this patient?

<130/80 mm Hg

His lipid panel shows that his low-density lipoprotein (LDL) is 140 mg/dL. What should you do next?

Counsel on diet and exercise. Start a statin. As a diabetic, his LDL goal is less than 100 mg/dL.

9. **A 45-year-old male with a history of HTN presents with acute onset of right knee pain and swelling.**

What is the differential diagnosis?

Gout, pseudogout, acute septic arthritis, bacterial cellulitis, trauma, Lyme disease

Knowing that he was recently started on hydrochlorothiazide increases the possibility of which diagnosis?

Gout

If you order a uric acid level and it is normal, does this rule out gout?

No. The level may be falsely low during an acute attack.

Your working diagnosis is an acute gouty attack. How do you confirm your diagnosis?

Aspiration of the synovial fluid with visualization of negatively birefringent, needle-shaped crystals

10. **A young adult female presents with a 3-week history of bilateral wrist pain. On review of systems, she has only noticed mild gum bleeding and mild fatigue. Electrolytes are normal. WBC is 2.1, platelets are 109, and hemoglobin is 10.5.**

Given her arthritis and pancytopenia, you want to rule out systemic lupus erythematous. What tests should you order for this purpose?

Antinuclear antibody (ANA), anti-dsDNA, anti-Smith antibodies

Which of the immunologic tests best correlates with lupus flares?

Anti-dsDNA antibodies

She later presents to your office with a BP of 142/80 mm Hg. What lupus complication are you concerned about?

Nephropathy secondary to lupus

11. A 32-year-old G1P0 woman at 32-weeks gestational age presents for a routine visit. Looking through her labs, you notice that she is rubella nonimmune and HBsAg positive.

Should you administer the rubella vaccine at this visit?

No. Live vaccines should not be given to pregnant women (wait until she is postpartum).

What treatment should you provide to the baby at birth?

Hepatitis B immunoglobulin, first dose of hepatitis B vaccine

12. A 21-year-old woman presents to your office with a 4-day history of profuse foamy vaginal discharge.

What is the next step in the workup of vaginal discharge?

Pelvic exam, KOH and saline mounts, gonorrhea and chlamydia probe

You suspect trichomonas. What would you see on a saline mount of the discharge?

Motile, flagellated trichomonads

What medication do you use to treat the patient (and her partner too)?

Metronidazole

13. A 45-year-old healthy woman says she awoke with a "red eye." She denies pain or history of trauma. Examination: well-circumscribed portion of the eye is completely red without evidence of conjunctival inflammation. Vision is normal.

What is the most likely diagnosis?

Subconjunctival hemorrhage

What are the underlying causes of subconjunctival hemorrhages?

Subconjunctival hemorrhages may occur spontaneously or secondary to trauma.

What is the appropriate management of a subconjunctival hemorrhage?

They usually spontaneously clear within 2-3 weeks, so no treatment is necessary.

What should be considered if a patient experiences repeated subconjunctival hemorrhages?

Workup for a bleeding disorder

14. A 65-year-old patient presents with a vague history of joint pain, weight loss, scalp tenderness, and a unilateral headache associated with pain in the jaw when chewing.

What is the most likely diagnosis?

Temporal arteritis (aka giant cell arteritis)

What workup helps you make the diagnosis?

Careful physical examination for tender arteries or bruits, elevated erythrocyte sedimentation rate or C-reactive protein, temporal artery biopsy

Patients with temporal arteritis are at increased risk for what ocular problems?

Ischemic optic neuropathy, central retinal artery occlusion, paresis of extraocular movements, irreversible loss of vision

What is the mandatory treatment of GCA?

Start high-dose oral corticosteroids immediately, even though biopsy results are not available immediately

15. **A 70-year-old male presents to your clinic with his wife. She states that she has noticed changes in his memory for more than a year and says he has become more withdrawn, although the patient denies this. A depression screen is negative.**

    What is the most likely diagnosis?

    Dementia

    What percentage of patients has a potentially reversible form of dementia?

    15%

    What lab workup should you do to determine if the condition is reversible?

    CBC, electrolytes, thyroid function tests, syphilis test (VDRL/RPR), HIV test, B_{12}/folate levels, brain CT or MRI

    If the patient also complained of urinary incontinence, ataxia, and has dilated cerebral ventricles on imaging, what is the most likely diagnosis?

    Normal pressure hydrocephalus

    If all the tests are within normal limits, except for diffuse atrophy and flattened sulci on imaging, what is the most likely diagnosis?

    Alzheimer disease

16. **A 23-year-old G2 now P2 postop day two from a repeat cesarean delivery has a firm but tender fundus on examination. She also has fever, tachycardia, and foul-smelling lochia.**

    What is the most likely diagnosis?

    Endometritis

    What are other common causes of postop fever?

    Wound infection, atelectasis, urinary tract infection, venous thrombosis, drug fever

    What kind of antibiotics would you use to treat her presumed endomyometritis?

    Clindamycin plus an aminoglycoside (such as gentamicin)

    Why do you need clindamycin?

    Anaerobic coverage (cesarean section in close proximity to gastrointestinal tract)

17. **A 20-year-old male presents with an acute, painful swelling of the testicle, with fever, dysuria, and tender scrotal mass on examination.**

    What is the most likely diagnosis?

    Acute epididymitis

What other diagnosis is necessary to rule out in the setting of acute testicular pain?

Testicular torsion

What test do you order to rule out testicular torsion?

Scrotal ultrasound with Doppler

18. A 45-year-old man with diabetes presents with a "yellow toenail" involving the distal portion of his right big toe. He has no pain but does not like the way his nail looks. He joined a gym 4 months ago and says that he has not had any trauma to his foot or toes. You remove his socks (which are damp) and note that his nail is thick, brittle, and discolored. You do a subungual scraping and prepare the sample with potassium hydroxide (KOH); microscopic viewing reveals hyphae.

What is the most likely diagnosis?

Onychomycosis

What is the most likely infectious agent?

Trichophyton rubrum

What hygienic measures would you recommend to this patient?

Wear clean, breathable socks and change often (2-3 times a day) to keep feet dry; wear comfortable, breathable shoes; wear foot protection in communal gym showers; control blood glucose

In general, do topical antifungals effectively treat onychomycosis?

No

What oral medications are used to treat onychomycosis?

Antifungals, such as fluconazole, itraconazole, terbinafine. Note: use azole antifungals with caution if the patient is on a sulfonylurea for treatment of diabetes because of risk of hypoglycemia. Follow recommendations for monitoring of blood counts and liver enzymes.

19. A 40-year-old man presents to your office complaining of 4 days of lower back pain after he was moving boxes in his attic. Examination: Normal motor and sensory function of the lower extremities. Negative straight leg raise test. Tense paraspinal muscles in the lumbar region.

What is the most likely diagnosis?

Lower back strain

Are any diagnostic tests necessary to make the above diagnosis?

No

What is the treatment for lower back strain?

NSAIDs for 7-10 days; supportive modalities, such as heating and light stretching; muscle relaxants are occasionally indicated; also educate the patient on core strength exercises to help prevent future injury

20. **A 7-month old presents with a 2-day history of cough, nasal congestion, and fever (100°F). He has six wet diapers a day and is playful. Examination: Normal except for nasal congestion.**

What is the most likely diagnosis?

Upper respiratory tract infection

The patient's mother wants you to prescribe antibiotics. What do you do?

Do not prescribe antibiotics since this is most likely a viral etiology. This is a good opportunity for parent education.

He is not up to date on his vaccinations. In this scenario, is it safe to administer vaccines even though he has a fever?

Yes

21. **A 6-year-old boy presents with a sore throat and fever (102.5°F) but no cough or nasal congestion. Examination: Tender cervical lymphadenopathy, tonsillar erythema and exudates, palatal petechiae. He has no drug allergies.**

What is the most likely diagnosis?

Streptococcal pharyngitis

What is his Centor score and based on that score, what is your next step in management?

His score is four (you can add one more point for his age of less than 15 years but this does not make a difference in interpretation). Treat empirically for streptococcal pharyngitis. Also treat symptoms supportively (salt water gargles, pain medication).

What antibiotic regimen should you use to treat this patient?

Oral penicillin V potassium for 10 days or one time dose of penicillin G benzathine IM

If the patient's Centor score had been 2 or 3, what would have been the next step in management?

Perform streptococcal antigen testing ("rapid strep test"). Positive rapid test → antibiotics. Negative test → throat culture. In either case, treat symptoms supportively.

If the rapid test is negative, why do you need to obtain a throat culture?

A throat culture is much more sensitive than the rapid test. If the rapid strep test is negative, it is okay to wait for the culture results (antibiotics can be given within the first 9 days of infection and still be effective in helping prevent complications).

22. **A 49-year-old woman complains of irregular menses over the past few months as well as discomfort with intercourse (not alleviated by over-the-counter lubricants). Your review of systems also reveals that she has been feeling irritable and has been experiencing episodes of hot flashes (lasting a few minutes). She has always previously had normal menstrual cycles. Her physical exam is completely normal, except for some vaginal dryness.**

What is the most likely diagnosis?

Perimenopause

What is menopause?

Amenorrhea for 12 months due to normal aging or surgical removal of the ovaries

What is the average age for menopause?

51

During perimenopause, what happens to FSH, LH, and estrogen levels?

FSH and LH rise, estrogen falls

What kinds of food products have been shown to worsen hot flashes?

Alcohol, caffeinated beverages, spicy food, food high in saturated fat

For a woman who still has her uterus and has decided to try hormone replacement therapy, what additional medication should be given in conjunction with estrogen to help prevent endometrial cancer?

Progestin

The Women's Health Initiative (WHI) which looked at continuous estrogen-progestin treatment found that this therapy increases women's risk for what diseases?

Heart attack, breast cancer, blood clots, stroke

The WHI found that continuous estrogen-progestin treatment decreased the incidence of what health problems?

Bone fractures, colon cancer

What kind of medication could you prescribe to alleviate her symptom of vaginal dryness?

Intravaginal estrogen

23. **A 62-year-old female presents to you with 1 day of vaginal bleeding. She has been menopausal for 9 years.**

    Because she only had 1 day of vaginal bleeding, she does not need endometrial assessment. True or false?

    False. Any vaginal bleeding in a postmenopausal woman requires further evaluation.

    What is the differential diagnosis of vaginal bleeding in postmenopausal women?

    Atrophic endometrium, endometrial polyps, endometrial cancer, endometrial hyperplasia, hormone replacement therapy, cervical cancer, fibroids

    What are the first-line methods of assessing the endometrium?

    Transvaginal ultrasound and endometrial biopsy

    You order a transvaginal ultrasound, and the endometrial lining is 6 mm thick. What is the next step in the work up?

    Endometrial biopsy, which is indicated when the endometrial lining is thicker than 4 mm in postmenopausal women

24. **A mother brings in her 2-year-old son after witnessing a seizure that lasted 3 minutes. Earlier in the day, his mother noticed clear nasal discharge and documented a temperature of 101.1°F. This is his first seizure, and your physical exam is normal other than rhinorrhea.**

What criteria are needed to make a diagnosis of febrile seizures?

Convulsion with a temperature greater than 38°C (100.4°F), age less than 6 years, no central nervous system infection or inflammation, no acute metabolic abnormality, no history of previous afebrile seizures

How can you distinguish between simple and complex febrile seizures?

Simple febrile seizures last less than 15 minutes and are not associated with focal features; if they occur in series, the total duration is less than 30 minutes. Complex febrile seizures last longer than 15 minutes and have focal features; if they occur in series, the total duration is longer than 30 minutes.

Which vaccines can slightly increase the risk of febrile seizures?

DTaP and MMR

When is neuroimaging indicated for febrile seizures?

Presence of focal neurologic features or signs or symptoms of increased intracranial pressure

Will he be at increased risk for intellectual impairment following this febrile seizure?

No. Febrile seizures do not increase the risk for future development of cognitive deficits, intellectual impairment, or behavioral disorders.

25. **A 42-year-old man, who is accompanied by his wife, presents to you after an episode of loss of consciousness. Yesterday, while watching television, his wife reports that he was unresponsive and "staring off into space" for 3 minutes. Simultaneously, she noticed that he was smacking his lips repeatedly. Afterwards, he was more responsive but also confused and somnolent. He does not recall the episode but mentions that he remembers seeing flashing lights. His vital signs and neurologic exam are normal. He has never had seizures, is not on medication, and drinks 1-2 alcoholic beverages per week. His mother was on a medication for a "seizure problem."**

You think he had a seizure. How would you classify it?

Complex partial seizure preceded by a simple partial seizure

What conditions can cause new onset seizures?

New onset epilepsy, cerebrovascular disease, brain tumor, brain injury, alcohol or illicit drug use or withdrawal, infections (meningitis, encephalitis), fever (in children), medications, metabolic disorders (hypo- or hyperglycemia, electrolyte disorders, liver, or kidney failure)

According to the American Academy of Neurology (AAN) guidelines, what imaging tests should be ordered in an adult with a first unprovoked seizure?

An electroencephalogram (EEG) to provide information about possible recurrence and a head CT or MRI (an MRI is preferable) to reveal structural lesions

His workup was negative, and you initially decided not to start him on antiepileptic drug therapy. He is seizure free over the next 6 months but then presents to you after another seizure. You decide to start him on an antiepileptic drug. What are the goals of therapy?

Control seizures, avoid side effects, maintain/restore quality of life

What percentage of patients with new onset epilepsy will become seizure free with the first AED prescribed?

50%

What should you tell him about driving limitations?

Most states require a 3-18 month seizure-free period before a patient may resume driving; however, each state has its own specific regulations. (www.epilepsy.com/epilepsy/rights_driving)

26. A young woman presents with swelling, tenderness, and warmth over the nasal aspect of the lower left lid. You apply pressure to the left lacrimal sac and note a purulent discharge coming from her tear duct.

    What is the diagnosis?

    Dacryocystitis

    What is the treatment?

    Warm compresses, massage of the lacrimal sac, antibiotic ointments

27. A 24-month-old boy with a small umbilical hernia presents with his mother for a well-child exam. He is doing very well and has no worrisome symptoms. However, his mother is concerned about the umbilical hernia and wants to be referred to a surgeon. You examine the child and find that his hernia is easily reducible, and he has a soft, nontender abdomen. You are able to reassure the mother that the umbilical hernia is not currently causing problems and that it would be best to continue observation.

    The mother would like to know how long the hernia will be present. What do you tell her?

    While hernias often close in the first year, it can take 2-3 years

    When is surgical intervention of an umbilical hernia required?

    If it does not close on its own by age 4-5 years, causes symptoms (pain), or becomes incarcerated/strangulated

28. A 25-year-old female presents with right eye pain that has become progressively worse over 5 days. The pain is worse with eye movement and she also states that she has had blurry vision (worse when she went for a jog 3 days ago). During your exam, you move your penlight briskly back and forth from one eye to the other. You note that her right pupil constricts consensually when you shine the light in her left eye, but when you shine the light in her right eye, her right pupil initially constricts but then dilates. Her left pupil is normal.

    What is the most likely diagnosis?

    Optic neuritis

What autoimmune neurologic disease is associated with optic neuritis?

Multiple sclerosis

What is the term for the type of papillary response seen in this patient?

Relative afferent papillary defect (Marcus-Gunn Pupil)

29. **A 45-year-old woman with a history of anxiety and diabetes presents to the clinic desperately worried that she has suffered a stroke because she can barely move the left side of her face. She explains that she woke up with "crooked" lips and was unable to chew her breakfast well. Her left eye is dry because she cannot close it fully. She does not complain of vertigo. On exam, you confirm her description of symptoms and also note that she cannot wrinkle her forehead. There are no other neurologic abnormalities and she has no blisters in or around her mouth and ears.**

What is the most likely diagnosis?

Bell palsy

Which one of her chronic conditions is associated with a higher incidence of Bell palsy?

Diabetes

What is the treatment for Bell palsy?

Oral prednisone should be initiated as soon as possible after the onset of symptoms (preferably within 72 hours). Some evidence shows that 7 days of antivirals (acyclovir, valacyclovir) may be helpful. Instruct the patient on eye protection (lubrication, shielding from debris), especially at night, to avoid corneal abrasion.

Will a patient's symptoms resolve without treatment?

With or without treatment, permanent facial weakness is uncommon, and most patients recover fully in 3-6 months. In theory, treatment decreases the recovery time and also increases the likelihood of full recovery.

What single physical exam sign makes this patient's symptoms unlikely to be caused by a stroke?

The patient cannot wrinkle her forehead, indicating that she has a lower motor lesion. An upper motor neuron lesion, such as a stroke does not affect the forehead because innervating fibers stem from both cerebral hemispheres; the contralateral fibers cross at level of the brainstem.

If the patient had presented with severe facial pain, vertigo, and blisters on the pinna of the ear, what would be the most likely diagnosis?

Ramsay-Hunt syndrome (herpes zoster oticus)

The patient recalls developing a rash a few weeks ago shortly after a camping trip, and today, she also complains of arthralgias. What diagnosis would you add to your differential diagnosis?

Lyme disease

How does the time course of her symptoms make them unlikely to be due to a tumor?

A tumor would bring the symptoms on more insidiously

Recommended Websites

American Academy of Family Practitioners
http://www.aafp.org

American Congress of Obstetricians and Gynecologists
http://www.acog.org

American Diabetes Association 2010: Clinical Practice Guidelines
http://professional.diabetes.org/CPR_search.aspx

American Thoracic Society
http://www.thoracic.org/

Centers for Disease Control and Prevention (CDC)
http://www.cdc.gov

Infectious Diseases Society of America
http://www.idsociety.org/

National Initiative for Children's Healthcare Quality (evaluation of ADHD)
http://www.nichq.org/adhd.html

National Institute of Diabetes and Digestive and Kidney Diseases
http://www2.niddk.nih.gov/

National Institute of Health
http://www.nhlbi.nih.gov/

National Kidney Disease Education Program
http://www.nkdep.nih.gov/

The Seventh Report of the Joint National Committee on Prevention, Detection, Evaluation, and Treatment of High Blood Pressure (JNC 7)
http://www.nhlbi.nih.gov/guidelines/hypertension/

Third Report of the Expert Panel on Detection, Evaluation, and Treatment of High Blood Cholesterol in Adults (Adult Treatment Panel III)
http://www.nhlbi.nih.gov/guidelines/cholesterol/index.htm

United States Department of Health and Human Services: Agency for Healthcare Research and Quality: Guideline database
http://www.guideline.gov

United States Preventive Services Task Force
http://www.ahrq.gov/clinic/uspstfix.htm

Violence Prevention (CDC)
http://www.cdc.gov/violenceprevention/index.html

Women's Health Initiative
http://www.nhlbi.nih.gov/whi/index.html

World Health Organization
http://www.who.int/en/

Index